Psychotherapist and hypnotherapist S.... .... thousands of addicts in her clinics in London's Harley Street, New York, LA and Europe. She has over 23 years' experience and her clients range from A-list actors to rock stars and sports personalities. She accompanied the England football squad to the Japan World Cup and has made many TV appearances. She is also the author of *Hypnodiet*, *F*** Diets* and the Amazon bestseller *Stop Smoking in One Hour*.

Praise for *Hypnodiet*

'After the hypnotism, I want to go to the gym every day . . . I just want to get more toned and healthy. I've never been happier' Lily Allen

Susan Hepburn's Hypnodiet is 'the hottest body trend of 2009' *Grazia*

'The secret to Lily Allen's dramatic weight loss has been revealed – hypnotherapy . . . with Susan Hepburn' *Daily Mail*

'I didn't really feel like I was on a diet at all . . . I've learnt how to change the way I eat and I hope it'll stay with me for life' Beth McLoughlin, *Now magazine*

'Susan Hepburn has transformed Lily Allen's attitude to food and exercise . . . Thankfully you don't need to be a multi-platinum-selling musician to benefit from her 23 years of experience in hypnotherapy' *Observer*

'Lily Allen underwent hypnotherapy sessions with Harley Street hypnotherapist Susan Hepburn to re-program her brain to enjoy eating healthy foods and feel positive about exercising' *Daily Mirror*

Also by Susan Hepburn

Hypnodiet

HYPNOQUIT

HOW TO BREAK FREE OF **ANY ADDICTION** – FOR EVER

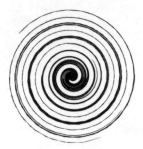

SUSAN HEPBURN

piatkus

PIATKUS

First published in Great Britain in 2011 by Piatkus

A CIP catalogue record for this book
is available from the British Library.

ISBN 978-0-7499-5233-4

Typeset in Sabon by M Rules
Printed and bound in Australia by
Griffin Press

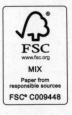

FSC
www.fsc.org
MIX
Paper from
responsible sources
FSC® C009448

Piatkus
An imprint of
Little, Brown Book Group
100 Victoria Embankment
London EC4Y 0DY

An Hachette UK Company
www.hachette.co.uk

www.piatkus.co.uk

Acknowledgements

I would like to thank all those wonderful professionals who have helped me to produce this self-help book; and my amazing family and friends for putting up with my continued absence, while I write and, most of all, I would like to thank all the people I have been able to help all these years to quit their addictions, because without them this book wouldn't have been possible.

Contents

Introduction

In over 23 years as an addictions expert, I have worked with thousands of people from all walks of life, helping them to overcome the addictions that are taking over their lives. Absolutely anyone can develop an addiction to almost anything. Each one of us is vulnerable and we have to deal with life's problems and our own issues, and it is these issues that sometimes lead us to depend on something – be it drink, drugs, shopping or smoking – to help us to get by. This can happen regardless of the life we are leading, whether we are a hedge-fund manager, a single mum struggling to cope with a young family or an A-list actor – we are all the same at the end of the day. So how do addictions start?

There may be numerous, complex reasons why one person feels compelled to take a break from the harsh reality of life and indulge in a different world through an addiction. For some, this is an occasional self-indulgence: they'll dip into it now and again, but it doesn't control them. Others, however, become hooked, and life then becomes lost in an addiction haze.

If this is you, and you truly want to free yourself from the grasp of your addiction, I have good news for you. You really can overcome your addiction with the help of hypnosis. I have helped people to break free from smoking, alcohol, chocolate, the Internet, work, shopping, drugs and many more. The case for hypnosis as a cure for addictions has been proven time and time again.

I began my career as a psychologist, but was drawn to hypnotherapy because I realised that hypnosis could bring about far quicker, longer-lasting results. I am aware of just how powerful the mind can be, and the combination of results plus speed fascinated me. I am a psychotherapist practising mostly in Harley Street, but I also travel the world helping people to cast their addictions aside.

Hypnoquit is a simple and effective way to free yourself from addictive behaviour. I call it a 'mind-changing revolution', because it works quickly, effectively and from the inside out. Don't worry, though, I'm not going to ask you to enter into therapy, or cope with blame or anguished soul-searching. Instead, I will simply help you to remove the guilt, anxiety and stress that is associated with your addiction. You will then build patterns of behaviour that are completely free from cravings.

There is, however, one important caveat. Hypnosis will only work if you are genuinely motivated to quit for you *alone*. You have to want to give up your addiction *for yourself* and not because you are being pressurised by someone else to change. If you can confidently say that this is true, then the rest is plain sailing. Using this book and the accompanying CD will quickly and easily help you to change your destructive patterns of behaviour. You will recapture your self-confidence and rebuild healthy and normal relationships.

You will never look back.

If you are now thinking, *but I've tried other methods before, and failed. Why should this work?* you are not alone. I often see people who say they have tried everything possible and that they have come to me as a last resort. They may even have been in and out of rehab numerous times. These people are often at the end of their tether and in total despair – and often their loved ones are too. But I always tell everyone who comes to me for help that this isn't just another try. This is the end of the addiction.

So, why should they, or you, believe me? Conventional methods of therapy for addiction tend to fuel anxiety and guilt. This is why they invariably don't work in the long term. But with Hypnoquit, I help you to remove the guilt and anxiety. What's more, there are no rehab centres, no halfway houses and there is no deprivation. Instead, using simple daily exercises, I am going to help you to 'reprogram' your mind so that you make long-lasting and life-enhancing decisions.

> There is no 'deprivation' with Hypnoquit. The change comes from within you, using the power of hypnosis to change your mindset.

With this method, your entire relationship with your addiction changes. As you begin to understand it, perhaps for the first time, you will want to make active changes, and you will quickly begin to behave in a different, more healthy and sustainable way.

★ **Case Study:** Colin, 31, is an IT expert who was addicted to smoking.

Before treatment:

'I smoke whenever I can during the day: when I get off the bus, walking to work, drinking with friends, chilling out after work. I smoke all evening and have been known to wake up during the night for a smoke.

'I am totally addicted to smoking and have been since I was 12 years old. I avoid going abroad other than visiting my parents who live overseas, as I can't bear the thought of being irritated and craving a smoke while on a flight. My father is too ill to travel, as he had a triple heart bypass because of smoking. I have to use patches and Nicorette gum just to get me through the flight.

'I feel old and tired. My best friend recently died from lung cancer and I thought, Why am I smoking, I can't believe I am doing this to myself? I am unhealthy, overweight and have a poor diet, and yet I am still smoking. I have got to stop. I am very unhappy and feel totally negative.

'A friend told me about the Hypnoquit method and how easy it was to quit smoking with none of the usual withdrawal symptoms. She said that she felt more positive about life after the treatment, so I decided that I would give it a go. What have I got to lose? I want to make life changes for the better and I want to get my confidence back.

'I lack energy and motivation to go to the gym, which is hardly surprising, as I can easily smoke over 20 a day.'

After treatment:

'I have not wanted a cigarette at all. It's as though I have never smoked. Strangely, everyone I see smoking I feel sorry *for, and I think how silly they look. I've had no withdrawal symptoms. It did seem strange at first, and I was waiting for the snacking to start, but to my amazement it didn't. I am very happy and have already joined a gym. I tried so many times to quit smoking, and gave in each time because I was bad tempered and I didn't like myself or how I was feeling. This has been so easy and I feel clean and healthy; I can taste my food and I am delighted.'*

WHAT IS HYPNOSIS?

When you say the word 'hypnosis' most people think of trances or gimmicky TV shows in which a Svengali-type figure 'controls' what you do. This could not be further from the truth. I never 'put people under' or play tricks on their mind. In fact, you would not allow me to, even if I could. What's more, with hypnosis you always remain in control. I simply use it as a form of deep, but lucid, relaxation to enable the changes to be made.

When you are in the deep and relaxed state of hypnosis, your heart rate, breathing and metabolism all slow down. Studies show that there are changes in brain activity too. In this altered state of consciousness you have an increased ability to listen and communicate. Your natural resistance is gone, and you organise your thoughts more clearly.

Crucially, when you are in this relaxed state with no resistance, hypnosis can bypass your conscious mind, enabling me to reach the highly 'suggestible' subconscious. I then place agreed suggestions into your subconscious mind, such as overcoming your addiction. It's that easy.

The subconscious part of your mind is the part that governs urges and impulses. Studies have shown that because hypnosis reaches this part of the brain it is a hugely powerful behavioural tool. (In fact, there are well-documented cases of people using it to undergo surgery without anaesthetic.)

In your state of deep relaxation you will effectively 'delete' the triggers, emotional associations and thoughts that caused your addictive behaviour in the first place. It's rather like deleting files from a computer. You delete your negative triggers and associations and then reprogram your mind with positive, life-enhancing thoughts and behaviours.

I will teach you how to visualise your new life, free from addiction. Visualising yourself in this liberated new state will become part of your daily meditations. You will also use affirmations – simple sentences that you repeat to yourself – to reinforce the changes you are making.

Finally, with this method, I will ask you to keep a daily journal, where you will note down your emotions and physical sensations. It will help you to understand how your mood affects your addiction and vice versa, and you will be able to see daily improvements in your state of mind, your self-confidence and self-esteem. Your journal will help you identify your low points and your triggers. It is a simple, but vital, tool in quitting your addiction.

HOW MUCH TIME WILL IT TAKE?

You need to set aside just 20 minutes a day to listen to your CD – that's all. Even the busiest, most stressed-out person can find this small amount of time in their day. We all have busy lives and enormous 'to-do' lists, but don't let listening to your hypnosis CD be at the bottom of yours. If you say to yourself, 'I'll do it later' you probably won't. But if you set aside a regular slot for your meditations, it will become easier and easier. You will soon begin to look forward to this valuable 'me time'. Putting the CD on your iPod or MP3 player will allow you to continue your sessions even while on business travel or vacations.

As you do your daily meditations, you will replace your self-criticism with self-acceptance. Your self-esteem will soar as you begin to see what you can achieve, and how painless that is. Very soon, you'll find that you no longer crave the substance or behaviour to which you are addicted. For some addictions, such as smoking, one session is all that's required.

Case studies throughout the book will introduce you to people whose lives have been dominated by their addiction, causing ill health, great unhappiness, destroying relationships and often creating debt in the process. Those people have all been helped to start a new life free of addiction, and their experiences will give you encouragement to take that first step.

HOW TO USE THIS BOOK

Read all of Part 1 so that you understand about addiction and how you have become caught in its grasp. It also explains what is 'normal' and how hypnosis can help you to find normality again.

Part 2 describes the different addictions. You may only wish to read the chapter that is relevant to your particular addiction, but you would be surprised how many people discover that they have more than one addiction when they look a little deeper. I therefore suggest you read through the whole part when you can.

The beginning of Part 3 is aimed at the person or people who will be supporting your work towards quitting. The part then goes on to describe how, through your meditations, I will find the root cause of why you became addicted and delete it from your subconscious mind, and how you will begin to reprogram your mind through Hypnoquit. Chapter 16 brings all the suggestions from the book together in an action plan to help you to get started. The final chapter prepares your mind for the benefits of Hypnoquit and encourages you to begin your new life without addiction – now.

This isn't magic. There are no tricks. It's the simplicity of my method – tapping into the power of your mind in order to place required suggestions – that makes it so appealing and effective.

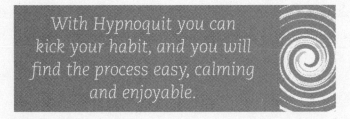

With Hypnoquit you can kick your habit, and you will find the process easy, calming and enjoyable.

Feeling trapped in an addiction that is controlling your life will be a thing of the past. The new you begins right here, right now.

Susan Hepburn

PART 1

YOU CAN QUIT YOUR ADDICTION

1

ARE YOU AN ADDICT?

How do you know whether you are addicted or not? First, let's look at what addiction is.

An addiction is a compulsion to engage in a specific activity and to repeat this activity time and time again, as if powerless to stop. An addicted person will either use a substance, or persist with certain behaviour, in order to feel good (or to avoid feeling bad). The compulsion can be so immense that they often go to great lengths to fulfil it.

Astonishingly, around one in three of us suffer from an addiction of some kind, but addictions don't all work in the same way. Drugs, alcohol, chocolate and nicotine, for example, all affect the way you feel, both physically and mentally. You then crave more of that feeling. Other addictions, such as shopping, the Internet or sex, give you a mental 'high' followed by a strong urge to do it again.

Of course, not everyone who enjoys shopping (or the Internet, or sex) is an addict – far from it. You may tick many of the boxes in the questionnaire on page 93, 'Are you a compulsive shopper?', but not be addicted. You simply enjoy shopping and may feel a little guilty now and then for over-spending, you may return a dress because you have changed your mind, but it doesn't make you a shopping addict. So, to clarify, if shopping dominates your thoughts – and you tick all the boxes – and you always get a 'high' followed by anx-iety and self-hatred, if you repeatedly buy the same items and definitely do not need them, then you are most likely a shopping addict. The same applies to Internet use and sex: if you are using the Internet to extremes, or your desire for sex is out of control and causing unhappiness, you have a problem. All these addictions will be explained in full in Part 2.

THE HIGH THAT TURNS TO A LOW

Addictions all initially give you a buzz, but this eventually turns to angst. This is the stage that you are at right now, otherwise you wouldn't be reading *Hypnoquit* (unless you are reading it out of pure curiosity).

Now that you are past the buzz stage, you need your 'fix' – whether it's chocolate, a cigarette, a prescription drug, a visit to the shops or alcohol. You feel that you need it just to func-tion and to feel normal. Although you may or may not have physical symptoms, there will certainly be mental agony if you deny yourself. This leads to a sense of powerlessness and despair. Your feelings towards that habit have now changed. When the addiction initially took a hold of you, it seemed amazing: 'Wow, why didn't I do this sooner?' Now you realise it's capable of destroying you.

★ **Case Study:** Jennifer, 19, was addicted to food and chocolate.
Before treatment:

'I became aware of the whole concept of weight when I was
13 when one of my friends said, "You would be really pretty if
you lost some weight." I felt embarrassed and wounded.

   'My sister is two years younger than me, but she gets all
the attention, because she is thin and has a nice body and is
outgoing, whereas I am quite shy. I get really annoyed, as my
mum and my sister are really close and they seem to laugh a
lot together and mum will say to me, "You are so serious
Jenny. If you lose some weight you will be happier and see life
differently, why can't you be like your sister?"

   'I started starving myself . . . one day I would hardly eat
and another day I would binge and make myself sick. There was
no pattern to this; it simply depended on my mood. I got thin
and thought I looked good, but my self-esteem was really low.

   'I was trying some jeans on and my best friend said, "Ooh
you look really lovely and skinny," and it stuck in my head.

   'My best friend and I used to share a meal sometimes or
decide not to eat dinner at all. I absolutely loved chocolate and
was not prepared to give that up, so I always ate my
chocolate in secret. I know I'm addicted, but I don't care.

   'I feel I have lost my childhood, I feel I never had a
childhood. I hate exercise and I feel that it is a punishment.

   'My mum told me about Hypnoquit and I was reluctant
at first, and then I thought, What have I got to lose? And it
gets my mum off my back.'

After treatment:

'I am surprised how this method has changed my whole
concept of food and addictions and has given me more time to

*enjoy other things in my life, like family, friends and sport.
Before hypnosis I never stopped thinking about food and
chocolate. Now I am so surprised that I am almost indifferent
to food, and I am so busy I hardly ever think about it unless
I'm hungry, which is a revelation in itself; I never knew what
it was like to be hungry before, as I was constantly grazing.
I do have chocolate now and again, but it doesn't have the
same buzz, it's just enjoyable. My sister and I are friends
now and I no longer think my sister is my mum's favourite.
I am doing better with my studies and I do see a purpose in
life now.'*

WHO BECOMES AN ADDICT?

Anyone can develop addictions and dependency problems.
They are not limited to a certain age group, gender or income
bracket. But the experience of addiction is different for everyone. This is because there are so many factors in the mix: your
personality and disposition, your life circumstances and the
substance or behaviour to which you are addicted.

There is a common perception that an addict must be
'weak' in some way, but this is simply untrue. I have seen
people from all walks of life with dependency issues. Some
of my clients are extremely influential people; some of them
are successfully heading major public companies by day,
but their world changes by night because of their addiction.
Outwardly, they seem to have it all. They may be incredibly
successful, beautiful, powerful and high-profile people and yet
still they have become addicted. Of course, some people have
more disposable income to enable them to indulge; others,
however, have more spare time: they may be waiting around

for the next movie offer – or they may be unemployed because of the effects of their addiction. There can be any number of reasons.

How is addiction affecting you?

The actual experience of addiction is different for everyone. But I have found that all addicts have one thing in common: their dependency invariably damages their life. It harms their relationships, their career and their self-esteem.

Does this ring true for you? Are you suffering from the loss of your career due to your addiction? Or is it coming between you and someone you love? Or is it simply something that you would just like to remove from your life because of the money it costs and the time you spend thinking about it rather than thinking about other things?

Of course, not everyone is badly affected by their addiction – a social smoker is one example, and you may be one of them. But you know that you are hooked and you want to quit, partly for health reasons but also because most of your friends have probably quit already.

However bad your addiction feels you still go back for more, time and time again, because of the addiction haze surrounding you. You think you will never overcome your addiction and get out of this mess.

*Life is not meant to be lived
in an addiction haze.*

WHY DO PEOPLE BECOME ADDICTED?

Many addictions are simply the cigarette smoking that grew from the occasional one enjoyed when socialising, the bar of special chocolate that you looked forward to at weekends, or the glass of wine you drank to unwind after work. Others, however, are more linked to the desire to find a space that frees your mind from difficult feelings. There can be many complex reasons why someone feels compelled to take a break from the reality of life and indulge in an almost fantasy world: relationship issues, life's stresses, boredom, peer pressure, childhood trauma and even a genetic predisposition. For some, this break from reality is a mere self-indulgence, taken now and again, but for others certain factors dictate that they are more likely to become hooked.

When you indulge in an addiction such as cocaine, for example, the euphoria you get from this drug takes you into an unreal world, a blissful state, an 'Alice in Wonderland' moment – just like a fantasy – and for some the unreal world is scary and they either never go there again or they do so infrequently; others, however, become hooked.

> Hypnoquit will work for you whether you are, in your opinion, mildly addicted or severely addicted.

WHAT ARE THE EFFECTS OF ADDICTION?

Sometimes you don't believe you are addicted because you just see it as a habit. Smoking is one such example. You always smoke at particular times, and you might not see it as having a very detrimental affect on your life. Getting your 'retail therapy' is another. You don't feel that it's so bad that it is really creating problems. But, if you *have* to do those things regularly, you are, indeed, addicted and once addicted you will inevitably suffer financially, personally and, for many addictions, with your health. And those nagging fears are often at the back of your mind even when you are just classifying your addiction as a habit. Eventually, you want to rid yourself of those fears as you realise that this 'habit' has a greater effect on your life than you once thought. But when it comes down to it, giving up is not easy and you may have tried many times, failing each time and feeling more consumed by the guilt of your failure and your desperation to get out of this cycle.

The power of addiction

Addiction can be so powerful that it dominates your mind and affects your daily life and relationships, but it still has you going back for more. Some addictions can create a constant physical craving, where you are powerless to stop yourself and feel desperate and alone.

As an addict you will go to great lengths to score a 'hit'. If your addiction is antisocial or illegal, you may have to indulge in risky or criminal behaviour in order to satisfy your addiction. Although most addictions are not extreme, others might involve using dirty needles, interacting with dangerous unstable individuals, burglary, or any number of crimes to fund the addiction.

Many addicts are in denial and invariably will attempt to

hide their addiction. They begin to adopt covert behaviour as the addiction takes hold and they will hide their behaviour from others – drinkers hide their alcohol, smokers sneak cigarettes, food addicts eat in secret, drug addicts hide their drugs, heroin addicts inject between the toes, and so on.

Addictions affect not just your life but also the lives of those around you. When you are in the throes of your addiction, you ignore all your responsibilities and become selfish, as your hit becomes the most important thing in your life. You may even go on the missing list, causing your loved ones to worry about you, or you may find little time for personal hygiene.

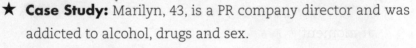

I will teach you to take control of your life and to no longer be addicted.

★ **Case Study:** Marilyn, 43, is a PR company director and was addicted to alcohol, drugs and sex.

Before treatment:

Marilyn lives in a cul de sac. Her neighbours are social animals – gathering in each other's houses for drinking parties in the winter and barbecues in the summer, with alcohol flowing. Initially, this only happened at weekends, but gradually they began to gather four or five times a week.

Soon, Marilyn became so accustomed to alcohol that she could drink two bottles of wine every night – party or no party. Her fitness-fanatic husband was frustrated with her. He could control his alcohol to an occasional glass of wine. Marilyn had gained over 12.7kg (2st/28lb) in six months. All resolve for healthy eating disappears under the influence of alcohol, and Marilyn was no different. She was eating takeaways, ice cream, pizzas and chocolate, and she regularly raided the children's treat drawer. She was dehydrated in the mornings and although she planned to drink water, she ended up drinking copious amounts of diet sodas instead.

Her husband was honest and direct. He wasn't the type to say, 'I love you whatever size you are.' He told Marilyn that he no longer found her fat body attractive and found it difficult to desire her sexually. He said, 'You need to get something done about it. You have lost self-respect by doing this to yourself, so how can I respect you?' But this made her defiant – so she drank more.

Then one day tipsy Marilyn was play-chasing with one of her children in the garden. Her daughter started screaming, saying, 'I don't like your voice Mummy and I want Daddy to put me to bed.' Marilyn was mortified. At that moment, she knew she had to get help. Her drinking was out of control, as were many other aspects of her life.

During our first consultation, Marilyn also admitted to me that she was addicted to two other things: prescription drugs and male prostitutes. She told me she'd been using male prostitutes for over ten years. She'd tried to stop when she had her children but she simply couldn't. It felt completely out of control.

She told me she'd wanted to try Hypnoquit years ago to cure her addiction to prostitutes, but was ashamed to admit it to anyone. I reassured her that whatever she could tell me about her addictions, I'd probably heard it all before – and sometimes more extreme versions – but, more importantly, the very nature of the addictions never occurs to me, as I'm not here to judge. I'm here to help.

After treatment:

Marilyn is now making excellent progress. She's eternally grateful to hypnosis. She has been free from all her addictions for 32 weeks now and is very confident that she will remain in this positive frame of mind. In the midst of her addictions, she just didn't seem to realise how much she had to lose. Now, with a clear head, she does.

WHAT DO PEOPLE BECOME ADDICTED TO?

People assume that addictions invariably involve alcohol or drugs such as nicotine. Although it's very common to be addicted to these substances, they are just the tip of the addiction iceberg. In fact, it is possible to become hooked on virtually anything.

I often treat people who have become addicted to sex, or to the Internet, to shopping, computer games, work, food, gambling and much, much more. Other less-known addictions, which have been treated equally effectively by hypnosis, are thumb sucking in adulthood, or men who have an addiction to wearing ladies' silk underwear. I have treated several men who need to wear rubber clothing and rubber boots during sex. If their partners are not interested and they want to stop anyway, Hypnoquit does help.

> *With Hypnoquit there is so little investment and yet the rewards are immense.*

You buy new shoes, win a bet, sleep with a stranger, swallow a pill, light a cigarette or drink a glass of wine, and you experience that high. Just for that moment, the world feels wonderful. You feel light, free, happy, 'better'. But as the high wears off, it's replaced by a yearning – the need to repeat the feeling. You may feel withdrawal symptoms – either physical or mental, or both. The urge to repeat the behaviour can become so powerful that it dominates your thoughts.

HOW DOES ADDICTION WORK?

Addiction doesn't happen overnight. Nevertheless, it seems to take you by surprise, and by the time you have to face it, you may have already lost control.

Addiction works in two ways:

1 **Physical addiction** happens when you take a substance, such as alcohol or drugs, which cause physiological changes in your body. When you use this substance it changes your body's chemistry. Used repeatedly, you can become physically dependent, and may crave the substance constantly. Without it, you experience withdrawal symptoms – often shaking, nausea, bowel changes, headaches and sleeping disorders. A physical addiction can develop through repeated use of prescription drugs such as antidepressants, tranquillisers

or sleeping pills. They all change the body chemistry, alter the mind and become highly addictive.

2 **Psychological addiction** is when you want, or need, your fix and you feel that you cannot function without it. The mind can become addicted to almost any activity that enhances your mood: addictions to shopping, sex, or the Internet all work this way. You experience powerful mental cravings. There are also often physical symptoms, such as anxiety, while you wait for your next fix, when you can repeat that particular behaviour until your mind is hooked on it.

> 'Every form of addiction is bad, no matter whether the narcotic be alcohol or morphine or idealism.' Carl Jung

WARNING SIGNS

Do any of the following apply to you?

1 Do you feel unsettled at the thought of quitting your habit, and would you prefer to quit later, say next month?
2 Do you become defensive if anyone suggests your habit is a problem?
3 Is your habit an important part of your life?
4 Do you spend most of the day thinking about your habit, and wanting to do it as often as possible?
5 Do you indulge in your habit to change the way you're feeling, or is it a compulsion you find difficult to do without?

6 Is your habit your guilty secret?

7 Do you often indulge in your habit on your own?

8 Do you need to have more and more of it to get the same buzz?

9 Have you ever tried to quit and been unable to do so, even though you know it's interfering with your career, your family or your relationships?

10 Has anyone asked you to 'Please get help'?

Prescription medicines, alcohol and drugs

If you are taking antidepressants or tranquillisers, or are seriously dependent on alcohol or addicted to hard drugs, it is essential to seek medical advice before using *Hypnoquit*.

★ **Case Study:** Rachel, 35, works for a documentary film company and was an alcohol abuser.

Before treatment:

Rachel is single and works long hours, socialising late into the night with other single 30-somethings in the city where she lives.

'I didn't start drinking alcohol until I was in my late twenties and only when socialising. All my friends at university were drinking copious amounts, but I just wasn't interested. I changed jobs and met a great bunch of people. Most of my friends were married with kids, so it was such a relief to find people my age, without ties, who were having fun. We'd go to bars, sometimes clubs, or restaurants. I didn't really like the taste of alcohol, but in no time I'd have two or three large glasses of wine, maybe some cocktails too.

I only actually got so drunk that I fell over about once a month, but I'd be drinking consistently: large pub measures, wine, cocktails or champagne. I would simply fall in with whatever my new friends were having. They would also have the occasional line of cocaine, so I did too. However, I began to notice this habit was becoming more regular. On my nights in alone, I'd open a bottle of red wine, order a takeaway and watch TV. My mind would wander to how great it would be to have a line of cocaine too, and it would make me feel less lonely.

'Often, I'd finish off the bottle late at night on the sofa and, I'm ashamed to say, I would sometimes fall asleep and wake up cold around 2.00 a.m., just as my father used to do. But I hardly ever felt hung over. Sometimes I'd go on a detox and not drink at all for a few days, or I would take myself off to a health farm and listen to like-minded individuals who were following the same pattern of behaviour as I was.

'But it didn't last long – this promise to myself of a "new me" – oh no, not much longer than a few days, and I would soon be going out again and I'd have to drink. Everyone was; it was part of the lifestyle. A friend and I were comparing and counting the units we drank in a week and I realised I was regularly consuming 40 or 50 units of alcohol a week – way over the recommended limit. That didn't stop me, I thought I knew better and even found it amusing that I could drink so much. We began to have drunken hysterical drinking competitions . . . until one day, I overheard someone say that I was a "cokehead and a drunk" and I was lucky to keep my job, and it came as no surprise that I was single. I was totally devastated – I had to stop this behaviour and I had to do it right now.'

After treatment:

'Hypnoquit helped me to turn my life around. I didn't feel that I needed to change my job or move away, as I felt confident that I could easily never drink alcohol again. Cocaine was no problem either, as that only ever accompanied alcohol. However, I did decide to have a complete change and to move away. I don't think my drinking pals would want me around them anymore and, quite frankly, I didn't really want to be around them. I am having fun, but a clear-headed type of fun. I don't blame anyone but myself, but I don't dwell on the past either, I am moving forwards and really enjoying my life more than ever, and I couldn't have done it without Hypnoquit.'

Stopping completely or relearning to be moderate?

To break some addictions you will have to stop completely. Smoking is an example. For other addictions, however, you will need to change your relationship so that whatever you were overloading on can be part of normal living once again. Food, for example, is essential to life, so you need to relearn how to eat in moderation. You can also learn how to use the Internet sensibly and to shop for things you need rather than buying for its own sake.

ARE YOU READY TO START?

Addiction can be scary and confusing. You may feel guilty, despairing and exhausted. You've taken the first huge step towards breaking free and finding a life without addiction.

Now, ask yourself if you are ready to begin. If you are not quite ready to quit right now, start an addiction diary. It will give you a clearer idea of what keeps your habit going.

EXERCISE: keep an addiction diary

If you are not ready to quit right now, it can help to keep a note of when, how and why you indulge in your habit.

1   Keep a small notebook in your pocket or handbag to use as your addiction diary.

2   When you feel the urge to indulge in your habit, write down how you are feeling, physically and emotionally, and what you are doing at that time. For instance, if you are addicted to alcohol, make a note of what you drank, where, and how much, and also how you felt at that time.

Your addiction diary helps you to build up a picture of how your addiction works for you. Every addiction is different. Usually there are emotional triggers that cause the impulse or urge. Keeping a note of your feelings at the time you get that urge can be enlightening. It helps you to understand your addiction, and therefore helps you to conquer it, from the inside out.

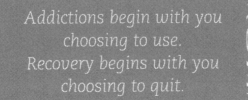
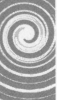

Addictions begin with you choosing to use.
Recovery begins with you choosing to quit.

I hope that this chapter has helped you to recognise that your addiction has far-reaching effects for your whole life, but all is certainly not lost. In the following chapter I will explain why it is that some people become caught in the trap of addiction whereas others keep control and, of course, I'll be paving the way to help you start on Hypnoquit.

2

HOW DID I GET
THIS WAY?

People often ask me, 'Why did I become addicted when others can take it or leave it?' There is no simple answer to this. In fact, there may be numerous, complex reasons. Addictions can start from a regular habit begun for no other reason than it was fun to do socially, like smoking occasionally or drinking in the pub with friends. Or it can be a well-earned rest from a day of hard work. But it can also be a way to temporarily lose ourselves from the problems we are faced with: relief from insecure feelings about ourselves as people, concerns about our relationships or our jobs, or a loss we just can't get over. In this chapter I'll discuss some of the situations that lead us to start and why some of us go beyond that occasional use to it becoming regular and heavier until eventually we're hooked.

IS IT TO DO WITH THE GENES?

You may have family members with addiction problems, and there is evidence that addiction can be genetic. No one is born an addict; however, according to various scientific studies, there are many ways that genes could cause one person to be more vulnerable to addictions than another. Likewise, it may be harder for people with certain genes to quit their addiction once they start. But someone's genetic make up will never doom them inevitably to become addicted. Environment plays a great role in addiction risk.

In research conducted by The University of Utah, Genetic Science Learning Center, mice were used to ascertain the gene factor in addictions because the return pathway in the brain functions in much the same way in mice as it does in people. So, to be a little scientific here, mice are leading the way in identifying addiction genes; for example, what is known as the A1 allele of the dopamine receptor gene DRD2 is more common in people with an addiction to alcohol and cocaine – hence the reason why these two substances frequently go hand in hand. It is certainly true that many of the people I have treated over the years have an addiction to both. Likewise, mice specifically bred to lack the serotonin receptor gene Htr1b are also more attracted to cocaine and alcohol. People with lower levels of the neurotransmitter neuropeptide Y drink more alcohol, and those with higher levels tend to abstain. Alcoholism is rare in people with two copies of the ALDH2 gene variation. According to study by Dr Hidetoshi Nakamura of Keio University in Japan (published in the journal *Thorax*, July 2003), people who carry the protective gene CYP2A6del allele are not good at processing nicotine causing them to feel nausea and dizziness. They don't get any pleasure out of smoking and therefore are less likely to become smokers. So, as you can see, your genes can play a part in your predisposition to addictions, but other factors such as environment have to be taken into consideration as well.

Other factors affecting children

There are many contributory factors why children become addicted to alcohol and drugs, with peer pressure being the single largest one. Also, there are environmental risks; if where you live, or where you go to school, has a favourable attitude towards drug use and alcohol, the risk will be greater for you to become addicted. Family can play a role too. If parents have drugs or alcohol around the home and are liberal – often sharing them with their children – those children could become addicted. The availability of drugs and alcohol, plus society's acceptance of them, is also a significant factor.

★ **Case Study:** Cassie, 29, is a mother of four small children and was addicted to alcohol.

Before treatment:

'My mother was an alcoholic. I remember, at the age of ten, pouring her bottles of vodka down the sink. I'd seen her out of control too many times and asleep on the floor where she had fallen. I thought I'd never be like that. My friends would come to my house to play and I would beg my mother to get up off the floor, as I felt so ashamed and didn't want my friends to see her like this. I was afraid they would tell their parents and then I'd have no friends. But they soon got used to my mother drunk, as it happened so many times, and they all found it amusing. I didn't.

'It's only now that I have young children myself, that I can see how awful it must have seemed to my friends. I'm embarrassed even after all these years. But I am more embarrassed that I too am getting drunk. At first, I felt in *control and I would say to myself, "There is no way I will be like my mother", but gradually it got worse and worse. It was a self-destructive thing. After a while, I just thought, Why not?'*

After treatment:
'I don't really know what I would have done without Hypnoquit. I do believe it has saved me, my sanity, my dignity and my self-respect. It has also saved my marriage, but more importantly this method has saved, and probably salvaged, my children's lives. They will hopefully grow up without any trauma or memories of their mum being on the verge of destruction.'

Cassie's situation is not uncommon, but sometimes there is no obvious cause for the addiction. It just happens. Many people never know or understand what drove them to become addicted.

As I explained in Chapter 1, none of this happens overnight. Addiction is insidious. People often tell me, 'It just crept up on me.' By the time they realised that they were addicted, it was too late to curb the behaviour without professional help.

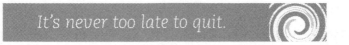

It's never too late to quit.

EMOTIONAL PAIN

Often people become hooked on a particular substance or behaviour because they are escaping from something painful in their past. Addictions invariably cause a person to lead a double life, which may include a well-respected professional life full of influential decisions, interacting with colleagues and leading a team, and an addicted life full of deceit, isolation, anguish, shame and self-disgust. If this is you, you probably feel those emotions are shameful and you want to change them but seem powerless to do so. Your isolation causes you to struggle to find happiness and your purpose in life. You question what life is all about and why everyone else is having fun when you are not. Your personal identity is challenged and you often don't see a way out. You become emotionally weak and can barely bear the pain.

> *Hypnoquit will help you to encompass self-love and personal growth, and to have the ability to feel emotional happiness instead of emotional pain.*

★ **Case Study:** Cheryl, 28, was addicted to prescribed sleeping pills and anti-anxiety pills.

Before treatment:

'My dad died when I was 14 years old and I was angry with him for leaving me. My mum says the anxiety started when my dad first went to the doctor's and thought he had cancer. I became lightheaded when he told me to prepare for the worst. My dad started popping pills to get him through the anxious time and was always at the doctor's. I suppose I learned the behaviour from him.

'Since his death, everything changed. I developed all

manner of health and mind issues and I'm always at the doctor's myself.

'I'm scared of so many things: I am scared of flying, of fast driving, especially on motorways, of heights. I am almost afraid of breathing. I'm getting married in August and I'm even worried about passing out on my wedding day.

'A few years ago I started taking sleeping tablets every night and sometimes I "doubled-up" and popped anti-anxiety pills too. Before I started Hypnoquit I couldn't begin to think of life without my pills. But my fiancé told me I had to come off them before we could start a family.'

After treatment:
'I started this hypnosis programme three weeks ago and already I feel immensely different. I used to worry about where we'd go on honeymoon and I wanted to control everything. Now, amazingly, I have just left it to my fiancé. I would definitely never have done that before. Also, I have not had one pill since I started the programme. I never will again – I just seem to know that for a fact.

'I feel I have made my peace with losing my dad as a child, and I am no longer angry. With Hypnoquit, my whole mindset has changed. I feel I have been set free.'

LOW SELF-ESTEEM

People often think that self-esteem means the same as confidence, but it's more than that. The Latin word for 'esteem' means 'to estimate', so in effect you estimate yourself. This short questionnaire will help you to 'estimate' yourself!

Questionnaire:
How good is your self-esteem?

	Yes	No
Do you like yourself?	☐	☐
Do you deserve happiness?	☐	☐
Do you deserve love?	☐	☐
Do you think you are a good person?	☐	☐
Do others like you?	☐	☐
Do you have some good friends?	☐	☐
Do your friends seem to enjoy spending time with you?	☐	☐

I'm hoping that your response will have been yes to most of those questions. If not, low self-esteem, along with other factors such as outside influences could put you at risk of addictive behaviour.

Pressures on the young

There are greater pressures in modern life to subconsciously compare ourselves to unrealistic stereotypes from the media. Young people often say they feel better about themselves when they have a few drinks of alcohol and can let themselves go; they feel more confident. Young people feel pressured to have to conform to exact ways of appearing in public: for women, perfectly groomed with designer outfits, styled and well-conditioned hair and manicured nails. And men too need to have perfectly groomed hair and nails and wear smart designer outfits.

Furthermore, there is no doubt that bullying in childhood

will have lasting effects on an individual's self-esteem which is invariably carried on into adulthood. Numerous studies have shown that bullies do not have self-esteem issues (as one would expect to be the case) whereas those who are bullied do. The bully is an aggressor and an abuser – often a 'ring-leader bully' (those who organise bullying) – and the bullied often live in fear every day of going to and from school, or play, or to take part in extra-curricular activities. They are repeatedly told that they are 'worthless' and that they deserve the treatment they are given. They believe it and their self-esteem plummets. Research has shown that long-term effects of bullying can be profound and include low self-esteem, a lack of self-confidence, unhappiness and increased problems with relationships.

Competition and stress in the workplace

The corporate world we now live in determines the competition among employees and their colleagues, senior management and their peers. People in their twenties and thirties in partic-ular are working very long hours and expected to produce ever greater results, working to achieve a bonus and to stay in jobs in the light of recessions and massive redundancies. They work hard and play hard. They often have heavy mortgages and become anxious if their expected bonus or salary increase falls below expectations. Hard work and exhaustion, partying to fit in socially with work colleagues, and being part of the team can also take its toll, as young people are increasingly very tired in the workplace, sometimes nursing a hangover. Working in a stressful environment can also have a big impact on your self-esteem.

Getting away from it all

Many people develop addictions as a kind of escape from the reality of life, a difficult situation, or even from themselves. A large number of my clients suffer from low self-esteem, even though outwardly they may seem incredibly confident and successful. An addiction promises you a way out: a way to escape from yourself, to feel more intelligent, more beautiful, more desirable and more competent. Although in reality, of course, it does the exact opposite: you spiral out of control, and your self-esteem plummets even lower.

★ **Case Study:** Ella, 49, is a TV executive and was addicted to alcohol.

Before treatment:

'I'm in charge of a team and a massive budget, I was recently promoted and am earning a fortune, but inside I feel like a fraud. I feel like I'm about to be exposed and that someone's going to come in one day and say, "What the hell does she actually do around here?"'

After treatment:

Ella started dating her 'Mr Right' (in her words) and she didn't want to mess this one up, as she had so many times in the past because of her behaviour after alcohol. She always became belligerent and 'ugly' and had been told this too many times. She was enthusiastic, and her enthusiasm enabled her to quit almost immediately. Ella was still alcohol-free after nine months and looked radiant.

STRESS

Pressure and stress are also common factors in addiction. I see many clients who were feeling absolutely fine until something difficult happened in their lives. This may have been unemployment that lead to poverty, or work stress, financial pressures, emotional strains, relationship break-ups or bereavements.

When you are stressed, you feel that you need to take refuge elsewhere – to take a break from reality. This life away from the stresses of reality can be associated with a certain substance or behaviour. It might just start with a drink in the evening, or smoking cannabis or taking cocaine, or even just indulging in your favourite chocolate. But over time, you find that you are relying on this refuge from day-to-day reality more and more. Before you know it, the reality break is controlling you, and not the other way round.

★ **Case Study:** Kevin, 35, is an IT engineer and was an Internet addict.

Before treatment:

'I started using the Internet just to unwind, and I would go online after a stressful day at work. I got into Second Life online, and it slowly took up more and more of my time: every evening, whole weekends.

'Unbelievably, I started calling in sick at work, because I wanted to chill out and go online. I felt I deserved it – my job was so stressful and I was being taken advantage of at work. My absence excuses became weaker and weaker.

'My boss soon called me into his office, which I knew meant trouble. He didn't really need to speak, as I knew what the problem was; his face said it all. "Kevin, there are lots of *guys out there who would love your job, so make changes or you're out. It's as simple as that."'*

After treatment:
'In these days of massive unemployment I knew this was serious, so I had to get help. I had bills to pay, and my life was going nowhere. That's when I decided to use Hypnoquit. I was very impressed with how quickly it worked. Almost immediately, I was able to use the Internet in my workplace and never use it at home. I simply have no desire to log on to Second Life. I listen to my hypnosis CD now and again if I feel a slight urge to use the Internet at home, but I don't think I really need to, it's probably me being extra cautious.'

Peer pressure is highly accountable for triggering an addiction, as is the social environment.

★ **Case Study:** Andrea, 30, works in advertising and was addicted to cocaine and alcohol.

Before treatment:
'I was at a party with my new boss and my colleagues, and the cocaine came out. Everyone was looking at me and challenging me, so I felt pressured to have a line of cocaine – and I loved it. I felt amazing, so confident. Everyone was doing it all the time, and it was free, as my boss always supplied it. He said it was our bonus for working so hard! I absolutely loved the cocktail of cocaine and alcohol, as I lost all my inhibitions and felt socially confident. The whole scene revolved around it after work, then I soon found a social scene that used it at weekends. Anyway, if I hadn't gone along with it, I don't think I'd have kept my job.

'I began to dislike it, though, and to become afraid of the long-term effects. The more I read and heard in the media about the long-term damage of cocaine use, the more afraid I became.'

After treatment:

'I am eternally grateful to my friend for introducing me to Hypnoquit – she had used it herself to quit her addictions. I feel like a new person, although I am probably the old me, just refreshed and without the addictions. I feel I have had a lucky escape.

'I am still in the same job and everyone seems to be continuing with their old addictions. I guess that I am not missed, as there is probably some other new executive taking my place. I don't mind at all, quite the contrary, as I am free. I realise that we have so many misconceptions about ourselves, about how others perceive us and how a possible outcome of a situation can be so wrong when you're looking at it through your addiction.'

Andrea's case shows that you don't have to change your job or your friends, for example, just because you have decided to quit your addiction. You are simply not 'doing it' anymore and you will gain strength through Hypnoquit to feel that you never have to bow to pressure, ever again.

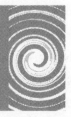

You will feel empowered and liberated, and you will realise that it's fun to not be addicted rather than the other way round.

HOW ADDICTION AFFECTS OTHER PEOPLE

I'm sure you are aware that addiction doesn't just affect your life. It affects the lives of those around you too: your partner, family, friends and colleagues. These are the people who care about you, or who work with you, and who worry about your health and safety.

These people may have to cover for you at work or at social functions. They may suffer on both an emotional and a practical level, because of your unreliability, your erratic behaviour and your changing moods, and they may be affected financially too.

Of course, you may be painfully aware of how your behaviour affects those around you, but you still can't stop yourself. Although you don't like to think of it in this direct way, the fact is you are effectively choosing the addiction over yourself and your loved ones. But you feel you don't have any choice at all, because you feel trapped, helpless and desperate.

★ **Case Study:** Allie, 45, was addicted to prescription drugs.
   Before treatment:
   'My husband would make excuses for me. At social events, he would say I was ill or exhausted – he'd explain away my sleepiness, or slurring – or my absence. He'd make jokes. He'd lie. It wasn't his fault – he was embarrassed and ashamed of me. Even now I feel awful, the pressure he was under was phenomenal. But in a way it helped me to keep taking the pills. He enabled me.'

   After treatment:
   'Of course, I do not blame him, but who can I blame? My parents? Sibling rivalry? Or even my peers? No, the buck

stops here with me. That's why I – the only one to blame – decided to get help. I also knew from talking and listening, when I wasn't too sleepy, that I had to find help for myself, and that no one could do it for me. Thank God for Hypnoquit, I say. I gave up all my drugs within five weeks. I was amazed, and I have no desire to go there again – and that was over one year ago.'

COMMON THREADS

Whatever their root causes, addictions invariably follow the same kind of pattern. At first you are in control of your behaviour, but gradually the 'feel-better high' you get when you indulge becomes more and more short lived, until you realise that it has taken hold of you. It dominates you. Often, you need more of the substance or behaviour to get a similar high. Eventually, it's not pleasurable anymore. It has simply become a need.

★ **Case Study:** Linda, 43, is a part-time teacher and was a shopping addict.

Before treatment:

'I ran up credit card bills of over £25,000 in just over four months. I managed to conceal them for ages. I felt sick with worry, though, and terrified of my husband finding out – I'd done it before, but never to this extent. I was also aware of the interest piling up on the credit cards, but I didn't know what to do. My husband is an accountant and he goes ballistic about paying extortionate interest. I was kidding myself that he would be cool about it once he got over the initial shock. I was so wrong. When my husband finally

found out, he was flabbergasted: total disbelief, then anger,
then a calmness and a distancing himself from me.

'Initially, he thought there'd been a mistake, and having
to tell him that there was no mistake was one of the worst
moments of my life. We didn't have much money and I was
working part time to supplement the family income. But I
was in fact spending my wages and some of his too. He said I
was totally irresponsible and selfish and he didn't know if we
would recover from this latest crisis.'

After treatment:

'Hypnoquit helped me to stop my shopping addiction
surprisingly quickly, almost instantaneously. I am not sure if
this is because I had too much to lose or because hypnosis
was so effective, but I do know that I certainly feel very
different this time from any other treatment I have tried, and
my husband says he has noticed the difference too.

'I haven't quite saved my marriage yet, but I am
working on it and feel happier than I have done for a long
time. We are still together, so there is hope. I know I'm now
free from my shopping addiction.'

WHATEVER THE CAUSE, YOU CAN
FIND RECOVERY

Here is the good news. With this method, it doesn't matter how
you got this way. I am not going to ask you to trawl through
your past looking for answers. You won't need therapy or endless hours of soul-searching and you don't need to blame
anyone, even yourself. You can put that behind you now.
Instead, you are simply going to reprogram your mind so that

you lose the urge to indulge in your addiction. It is fast, simple and easy.

In the next chapter I talk about what behaviour is normal and when behaviour gets out of hand and creeps towards addiction.

3

WHAT'S NORMAL?

Throughout this book, you will read many interesting case
histories, ranging from extreme addictions, such as people
whose lives are being overtaken by a compulsion to use the
Internet or by overeating, to normal everyday habits, such as an
addiction to smoking or drinking alcohol more frequently than
is considered healthy, which have no underlying causes other than
peer pressure. Some of the people in my case studies have learned
their addictive behaviour as a result of peer pressure, boredom
or perhaps childhood abuse in schools. I have heard many sad
stories of children who are given money in return for sexual
favours and are then led on to addictions to drugs, alcohol, smoking, pornography, and so on. With Hypnoquit I'm going to ask
you to put all that to one side. Whatever your addiction is, and
however it has developed, it is not part of the equation any more.
You simply want to rid yourself of it and to lead a normal life.

To do this, you will learn how to reprogram your mind using
Hypnoquit so that you no longer crave the substance or behaviour to which you are addicted. But before you can begin, you
have to *want* that normality in your life again, rather than
being pressurised by someone else to do so.

With Hypnoquit you don't need to relive your past. Put it behind you and look forward to a clear future.

REMEMBERING HOW TO FEEL NORMAL

Try to recall what 'normal' actually feels like, because often the whole idea of normality is lost when a person has an addiction. A normal relationship with your own urges and impulses is one that is free from guilt, fear or self-punishment.

When you are normal:

- You overindulge in treats now and again – such as chocolate, cheese, alcohol, or perhaps gambling on vacation – but you don't become angry or upset with yourself because of it and you may even find it amusing.
- You are able to say no, and mean no, when you feel you have had enough food, alcohol or whatever excites you or relaxes you.
- You are in touch with your body, making healthy choices most of the time, based on what you need to stay fit and happy.
- You are aware of your feelings and needs.
- You know your triggers – what drives you towards that escape from reality – and are able to decide whether to indulge or not.

★ **Case Study:** Deanne, 49, is a stay-at-home mother of two teenagers, who was addicted to food.

Before treatment:

Deanne has been addicted to food most of her life and, when she first came to see me, she was about 25kg (4st/56lb) overweight. She was miserable, desperate and tearful, and she badly needed help.

'I don't know if I even understand what it's like to stop constantly thinking about food: planning where, what, and when I'll eat next; shopping for food; for ever eating and only stopping when I'm asleep. I'm never hungry. I'm never full. I just desperately need to eat. I think about it all the time.

'I hate myself when I eat, but I can't stop. Food, and all thoughts about food, have taken over my life. I feel as if I can't really take an interest in other things, like my sons' football games, their exams, their school life. I'm just consumed by this yearning all the time, this feeling of emptiness and craving, these thoughts. They outweigh just about everything. I have no idea what it would be like to be any other way. I have no idea how normal people eat.

'I have to shop for my family day to day, because if there's food in the house, I will eat it. I buy something for me to eat while I'm cooking dinner – usually a sandwich, but I have been known to buy six cooked chicken thighs and eat those, plus a cake, while cooking. Then I eat chocolate and biscuits in the evening. Can you believe it?

'My husband never said a thing about my weight, so I didn't do anything about it. Then one of my children was crying when he came home from school. Other children had been teasing him on the way home, saying "Your mum's fat!". I had,

of course, seen people's faces when I sat next to them on planes –
and I've had the shop assistant telling me disdainfully, "There is
nothing in your size madam." But my child being upset gave me
the jolt I needed. I had used hypnosis before to quit smoking, so
this was the obvious choice for me. I had logged Hypnoquit in
the back of my mind, I guess subconsciously, for future use.'

After treatment:
'Hypnosis has worked for me and I am eternally grateful to
the wonders of the mind.'

Deanne felt 'mesmerised and intrigued' about how
quickly she started to make changes, from the first day of
her treatment. She also felt proud that she was introducing
her family to her new healthy-eating choices, and everyone
joyously agreed that they were tastier. Through Hypnoquit,
I taught Deanne to eat light, healthy foods and to avoid the
stodgy, sugary, starchy, salty and fatty foods she had been
used to having. The transformation was easy, as she was
convinced she would die young if she didn't alter her
eating habits.

MINDFULNESS CAN HELP YOU
RECAPTURE NORMALITY

A central concept of Hypnoquit is 'mindfulness'. It is a psychological discipline with its origins in Buddhism and it is becoming
increasingly popular as people search for a more serene and
thoughtful way to live in our hectic modern world. Clinical
studies have shown that mindfulness-based stress-reduction
programmes have been used effectively by mainstream psychol-
ogists to help patients with a variety of problems ranging from

pain management in cancer patients to relief from long-term depression. In my clinic in Harley Street, and when I travel to other countries, I use these techniques to help clients suffering with pain from cancer, arthritis and many other chronic conditions. Using those same techniques, I will encourage you to practise mindfulness in order to become more aware of your emotional and physical state and to recapture a sense of balance and normality.

This programme means that you will become more aware and in tune with yourself and your environment, and therefore learn to make more healthy choices for your well-being, both emotionally and physically.

When you live more mindfully – that is, you give the present moment your full attention, rather than focusing constantly on the future or the past – you will enjoy life far more than you do now. You will learn to live more calmly and to live in the 'now'. This means that you will find it easy to distance yourself from the cravings and triggers that cause your addiction.

> *As you do your meditations you will feel your body and mind relax, then we'll work together to help you to break your addiction.*

★ **Case Study:** Nancy, 45, is a nurse who was addicted to prescription drugs.

Before treatment:

Nancy came to see me because she was taking a large number of prescription drugs and knew she was out of control. She told me how her addiction had crept up on her.

'I worked as a nurse for over 25 years without being tempted to use drugs of any kind, even though I deal with drugs every day with my patients, and I have the key to the DDA [Dangerous Drugs Act] cupboard. Like all nurses, I work long hours in highly stressful areas, taking care of patients with horrendous injuries and dealing with tragic deaths.

'In nursing there is no grief counselling or briefing following a tragedy. There isn't time for it, and it's straight back to business. I see children dying, homicide victims, terminal illnesses and sudden deaths – all on a daily basis, with no emotional support, and I sometimes have to give emotional support to their relatives.

'I never gave it a thought because I was "tough". I would certainly feel sad and it would affect me, but the next patient was waiting, so there was no time to recover. But gradually I became depressed. I felt paranoid about my family and worried about something happening to my children.

'I had a friend who had told me several years earlier that she used some "leftovers" of the medication she gave patients and she said how great it made her feel. At the time I couldn't believe what she was telling me, and I almost felt disgusted with her. Well, a few years later, I found some "leftovers". I was having a hard time sleeping and I convinced myself it was OK, as it was just left over and I was only trying it out. The rest is history. The leftovers are in fact medication that should have been given to patients, but we would give them half their dose and keep some for ourselves.

'I never imagined that I would be in such a state, because I considered myself to be strong, reliable and principled. But I began to enjoy lying in bed, having a buzz and I liked being *able to sleep. I justified myself by saying it was just left over and my patients weren't suffering; they seemed OK.*

'Believe me, there were leftovers everywhere; I was like a kid in a candy store.

'Although I knew I was in trouble and needed help, I was terrified of seeking it, because I was certain that someone would turn me in to the state board. I was paranoid; however, eventually a deputy manager caught me, when my manager was away on maternity leave. I was reported to the professional body and suspended immediately.

'I have lost my nursing licence, and am awaiting disciplinary action, facing 40 counts for drug theft. I will also have a permanent criminal record, which will prevent me from working as a nurse or any other job in the medical sector, which is all I know. I am in a mess.'

After treatment:

'Despite all of this I have remained clean, and I plan to live my life without drugs, thanks to Hypnoquit. I really cannot believe the strength it has given me. I have become a grandmother and that has given me great joy: it's a distraction from the awful mess I got myself into. This programme not only helped me to come off the drugs but also to rediscover my inner strengths of self-confidence, self-esteem, self-worth and self-belief, and for that I am more than eternally grateful.'

HOW TO BECOME MINDFUL

So, how do you do this? Well, it's incredibly simple, although it may require some planning, and it will mean breaking some long-held bad habits, but the end result will make it all worthwhile.

As I've already explained, addictions are usually preceded by a trigger event, which sets off feelings and thoughts, and sometimes uncomfortable sensations. I use the word 'uncomfortable' here because you know it will lead to the urge to indulge in your addictive behaviour. Mindfulness gives you the tools necessary to take the time to think, so that you are aware of and recognise the triggers, enabling you to step out of autopilot and therefore stopping your addictive behaviour by taking back the controls. You are then able to take charge of your life, free from addiction.

> *Mindfulness can help you to make the decision to change your behaviour and your lifestyle.*

People often tell me that their urges and cravings seem to 'just happen'. But there is an unquestionable connection between negative emotions and addictive urges. With mindfulness, you develop an awareness of your emotions, and so you learn to anticipate, and bypass, your urges.

What is an urge and what is a craving?

An urge is a relatively sudden impulse to engage in a specific activity such as gambling or shopping. A craving is a desire to experience the effects of your addictive behaviour, time and time again, and it can exist for some time before you satisfy it.

CHECKING YOUR AUTOMATIC
IMPULSE WITH AWARENESS

Put simply, mindfulness is when your automatic impulse to snack or reach for another cigarette, an extra piece of chocolate, a line of cocaine or another glass of wine, is over-ridden by a more aware thought process, which says, 'No, I don't actually want any more, or 'I don't need it at all'. You are taking control in a positive way.

> Mindfulness teaches you to walk in the direction of healing and awareness, and away from the destruction of addiction.

Living more mindfully will help you to get in touch with how you are feeling – your urges, your cravings, your desires and needs. You will find that you can now listen to yourself at last. You can hear, anticipate and deal with your emotional needs and desires, rather than simply giving in and medicating them with an addictive substance or pattern of behaviour.

YOUR DAILY JOURNAL WILL HELP YOU

Keeping a daily journal is an essential part of Hypnoquit. It is a way of recording your feelings and your actions so that you can see how you are beating your addiction. Complete your journal as explained in Chapter 16 with your activities on one page and your emotions and behaviour on the other.

Each day, after you have listened to your CD, you will have written 'CD' in the top right-hand corner of that day's page in your journal.

As you complete each day's entries, you will begin to see a pattern emerging: you will start to see a correlation between the two entries: your feelings and your actions. You will also see, and be able to chart, your progress in quitting your addiction.

When can I stop the journal?

You will know when you no longer need to do your journal; however, you should keep it in a drawer so that if you need to refer back to it some time in the future, you will know where to find it. I suggest you stow it away somewhere with this *Hypnoquit* book. The only reason you may need to refer back to your journal – and this is highly unlikely – is if you find yourself slipping back into your old ways. Your journal can reassure you by showing you how you did it before, and where you have gone wrong now.

As you flick through the pages you will see clearly in the top right-hand corner CD – CD – CD – CD. This is your answer. Get back on track: listen to your CD.

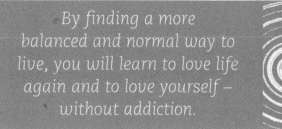

By finding a more balanced and normal way to live, you will learn to love life again and to love yourself – without addiction.

An example of a journal

Darian, 40, was addicted to alcohol and cocaine. Here is his journal:

Day one: 1st January 2010

Activities:

Started Hypnoquit programme today.

Kids are driving me nuts, as I want to do this and they want me to take them to the park to play football.

Exercise did me good – hour in park.

Enjoyed listening to the CD then off to bed, as we have early start tomorrow to go to in-laws.

Emotions:

Feel anxious about the programme, but promised Sandra I would do it on 1st January.

Feel slightly resentful and worry that I will miss out on something when my mates want to go to the pub and get some 'Charlie'. I can't . . . I feel anxious just writing this.

I've tried lots of ways to quit and nothing worked so maybe this won't either.

Did some soul searching today after a long chat with Sandra, who said I have a choice – 'Your family or your mates, it's as simple as that.'

I definitely want this to work.

Park with kids, I felt like a kid myself, as I have made my decision so was on a high just from realising that I don't need 'Charlie' to get a hit – my family give me that.

Day two: 2nd January 2010

Activities:

Up at 7a.m. for drive to in-laws. Crazy breakfast, kids yelling at each other. Me and Sandra yelling.

Fun day with in-laws, and always have lots of laughs. Kids happy to see grandparents too.

Yummy lunch.

Sandra giving me loads of grief over something I said to her Dad.

Mates wanted me to go out for a drink with them when we got back, but I said no. Put kids to bed while Sandra made dinner.

Did the meditation before bed, after dinner.

Emotions:

Looking forward to the day as in-laws are a good laugh and chilled.

Stressed during lunch with Sandra and still not sure why she was angry.

Wonder if Hypnoquit is going to work, probably not. Usually fail.

Tempted to go with mates – really, really wanted to. Wanted to go and let off steam, wanted a drink, a line, but knew it wasn't the right thing. Trying to be strong.

Pleased I stayed – reading boys a story felt right, and loving. I felt good about not going with my mates, afterwards.

Really calm after meditation. Feeling strong – but tired!

Day three: 3 January 2010

Out all day driving and visiting relatives. Long day. My little boy unwell, so really exhausted when we got back home late –so naughty me never did my diary! Hope this doesn't affect my progress.

Day four: 4 January 2010

Activities:

Out the door before breakfast – back at work!

Busy, busy all day, one thing after another, crazy day.

Clients for lunch. Asking tough questions, they're being tricky and evasive, quite aggressive.

Mates asking why I didn't go out last night – talking about club they ended up at.

Head down all day and got lots done. Said no to mates – again.

Home late, boys in bed but gave them a kiss. Dinner with Sandra.

Meditation last thing at night again.

Emotions:

Feel like I have energy for the first time in ages – enthusiasm for life. On way to work, smiling, feeling confident.

Less stressed, despite workload and difficult clients. Felt more able to cope. Calmer.

Feeling so strong. Was able to say to my mates that I am not interested in hearing about their night out. In fact, am going to spend more time with family, go out much less – felt really powerful, and in control for first time in ages. Beginning to think the programme is working!

Loved coming home to see boys before bedtime, happy at dinner with Sandra, we're getting on so well. I know my family is my 'high'. I don't need more. I can do this.

Meditation: totally calm afterwards. Really know this is going to work now. Feel no urge to indulge in my old habits at all. Just peaceful.

Making the right choices through mindfulness and visualisations

Mindfulness and the daily journal are essential parts of the Hypnoquit programme for any addiction. You will also help your mindfulness by using visualisations and incorporating affirmations into your meditations on the CD. In Chapter 15 I will explain all about making a Visualisation Tool, which is a picture of you without addiction. Around the edges of the picture you will write positive and meaningful statements (affirmations) that will help to reinforce your resolve to quit.

So, if you want normality, an addiction-free existence, a mindful approach to getting your life back, do your meditations and write in your journal every day.

That little book and the CD are more valuable than you can possibly imagine. They are your Hypnoquit toolkit. They will help you to rediscover what normality feels like, and to love your life again. With these tools, you will get your life back and learn to love and respect yourself again.

4

HOW CAN HYPNOSIS HELP YOU TO BECOME ADDICTION-FREE?

People often ask me how hypnosis works. They want to know how it can possibly free them from their downward spiral of addiction. I tell them, as I'm telling you, that it's a relatively simple, fast and straightforward tool that changes your behaviour from the inside out. But how exactly does it do this?

THE ASTONISHING POWER OF THE MIND

Hypnosis is defined as a state of deep relaxation within your body and a state of increased and heightened awareness within your mind. For years, hypnosis has caused intrigue, and it still does to this day. But the misconception that hypnosis 'messes with your mind', and that you will never be the same again, is simply not true.

It is popularly believed that hypnosis is a state resembling sleep and almost unconsciousness. This is a myth, and scientific research has proven time and time again that hypnosis is actually a wakeful state of focused attention, and heightened awareness and suggestibility.

In fact, hypnosis is one of the most powerful states for personal development and positive change. It allows you to access your creative potential. This is how all those long-held thoughts, beliefs and patterns of behaviour can be deleted and rewritten, if necessary. It isn't magic; it's the astonishing power of the mind.

Over the years, people have often asked me why participants in hypnotists' stage acts are asleep during the performance – after all, they look like they are asleep, their head lolls to one side and they seem 'out of it'. Yet clients in my room, or people who write to me after using my method through CDs or DVDs ask, 'Is it going to work, as I'm not hypnotised? I am awake and I could have opened my eyes at any time.' Well, with hypnotism you *are* awake. You are just deeply relaxed. Unless those stage-show participants were actually sleepwalking (which is highly unlikely), it is physically impossible to be in a period of activity, as they clearly are, while you are sleeping.

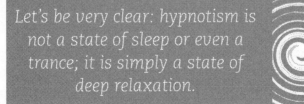

Let's be very clear: hypnotism is not a state of sleep or even a trance; it is simply a state of deep relaxation.

Just to reassure you, you *will* be hypnotised with Hypnoquit, even if you don't feel as if you are. You will be fully aware the whole time and you will enjoy the experience and achieve your results simply by listening to the CD. There is always this

misconception about hypnosis and trances or sleep-like states –
and it is a misconception that I have no doubt will continue for
years to come.

> **To avoid confusion**
> Hypnotherapy is simply hypnosis that is used for
> therapeutic reasons, hence the name 'hypnotherapy'.

 HYPNOQUIT tip

Motivation

Hypnoquit is a tool that will help anyone who has decided for
themselves – rather than being pressurised by a critical friend,
partner or parent – that they would like to be free from addiction. If
you think you're fine the way you are, but are only doing this
because your partner says you need to quit, and your resistance is
gone, then you may well struggle. Hypnoquit is something you
have to do for yourself. The good thing is, though, that anybody
who is truly motivated can use this method to rid themselves of their
addiction and to live a healthy, happy life. In most cases people
do not need rehab to do this.

HOW HYPNOSIS WORKS: DELETING
NEGATIVE THOUGHTS

Hypnosis works by short-circuiting – or deleting – negative
patterns of thought or behaviour. The effect can be felt in a
short period of time, and sometimes instantly, depending on the
addiction. Smoking is one negative pattern that can often be

deleted instantly. This is why I use the same analogy as deleting defective files from a computer: instant. Hypnoquit allows you to short-circuit all those negative thoughts that fuel your addiction: the self-destructive messages about yourself that you have absorbed over the years and the many times that you have tried to give up and then failed.

The Hypnoquit programme is not a cure for years of unhappiness or abuse, and it won't change our culture. It is simply a way to bypass all those unhelpful thoughts and impulses which cause your addiction, replacing them with new, healthy patterns of behaviour. Through deep relaxation, and reprogramming the mind, using your daily meditations and visualisations on the CD, you will be able to short-circuit your addictive behaviours.

With addiction comes guilt, anxiety and stress. Even though you know you should quit your addiction you can't, so the weight of guilt can bring tremendous feelings of anxiety and stress. This can also become an obstacle in seeking help to quit, because you feel unable to look deeply into the problems that caused your addiction and also the problems your addiction has caused. With Hypnoquit you will not need to revisit the reasons for your addiction or the pain they are causing, I will simply help you to remove these feelings associated with your addiction so that you can build patterns of behaviour that are completely free of guilt, cravings and addiction.

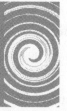

You will feel your body and mind floating into deep relaxation and peacefulness – leaving your cravings behind you.

DOES IT WORK FOR EVERYBODY?

You may well be thinking that it will never happen that way for you. Well, the first thing to understand about hypnosis is that virtually everybody has their doubts about whether it will work for them – or indeed, for anyone! I can assure you that Hypnoquit does work, and it will work for you too, even if you are sceptical, as Peter was, below.

★ **Case Study:** Peter, a 38-year-old banker, was addicted to alcohol and cocaine.

Before treatment:

Peter had a hectic schedule and worked long hours. His alcohol consumption was out of control, and he was not only punishing his body by drinking into the small hours and getting up early in the morning but he had also started to use cocaine. He felt he couldn't function any more without the combination of the two.

When he came to see me, he was sceptical, to say the least. But I could see that he was desperate too.

'I thought it was probably a load of nonsense to be honest. But I am desperate. I've tried addiction therapy, rehab, pills, willpower and going cold turkey. I've tried virtually everything going – been round the block – some things had worked for a few weeks, but I always end up back in the old, destructive, patterns of behaviour.'

His wife threatened to leave him and take their small children with her until he sorted himself out. He realised that she had had enough. They had been down this road too many times before. Other than providing money for them to live on, she questioned his usefulness in the family, since no one seemed to see him. On the rare occasions when he was around, he was either inebriated or prickly.

Something snapped, and Peter came to his senses and sought my help.

After treatment:

Peter is now well on his way to being in control of his life. He is a happy, laughing family man who now doesn't believe in looking back, only forwards. And somehow he knows he will never return to that dark time in his life.

WHY HYPNOSIS?

My career began as a psychologist and during my training I was fascinated by the hypnosis module; it really affected me, and it was as if I had suddenly found my vocation in life. I like the idea that results can be achieved incredibly quickly and effectively, and I knew that hypnosis was for me. After 23 years, I am continually passionate about my work and fascinated by how I can help each new person to bring about changes to their life.

I am often asked, 'Where do you get all your energy from?' Even my family has asked me this many times over the years. Well, I always 'practise what I preach', eating healthily and mindfully and making exercise an essential part of my everyday life and not an optional extra. Having a direction in life has many benefits too, including happiness and immense amounts of energy and, when you quit your addiction, you too will be happy and energetic as you find your direction.

Through all the years of helping people to conquer their addictions, I have yet to come across a treatment that is as equally effective as hypnosis.

Hypnosis is an amazing tool for change. Of course, not all hypnotherapy, or hypnotherapists, are the same. Many have different ways of working. Some are more effective than others, as in every profession, but the basic principles are the same. To describe how hypnosis works, it is often easiest to turn to the four most-common misconceptions about it.

Myth 1: I will be 'put under'

Many people think that when they are hypnotised, they will somehow lose consciousness – become zombielike and unable to control their actions. They also think that afterwards they might forget what happened – that the session would be a total blank. These are very popular beliefs, but they are wrong.

Fact With hypnosis generally – and certainly the kind I practise – you do not hand control over to me. The state of deep relaxation that you reach during hypnosis is known as REM (rapid eye movement) or the 'dream state' – a term you may have heard used for describing sleep patterns.

Hypnosis resembles the state you are in as you *enter* sleep: you are not fully asleep but you are not fully awake either, just very deeply relaxed. Because the body has slowed down, REM automatically takes place. (It is worth noting that REM takes place during the lightest part of your sleeping state and that you can easily be woken from this state; it is the state where the dreaming takes place. So, if you are woken during REM sleep, you will invariably remember your dream.) You get into that state purely by relaxing your body and mind, guided by my voice and my instructions. With Hypnoquit, you can do this at home, using the CD.

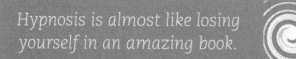

> Hypnosis is almost like losing yourself in an amazing book.

In this relaxed, guided state you will be calm but alert – more hyper-attentive than drowsy. You 'tune out' from everything around you but remain alert and focused. You can get up and walk away at any time during a hypnotherapy session. You can choose to ignore or blot out the whole thing, or you can choose to let it in.

In other words, hypnosis is not something that's done *to* you – it's something you do *for yourself*. It stands to reason, therefore, that the more motivated you are the better Hypnoquit will work for you.

Myth 2: some people just can't be hypnotised

Most people, during their first session, think it's not working. They feel wide-awake, fully conscious – even critical – and assume that this means they are in some way resistant to the method (or that the hypnotherapist is having an off-day!).

Fact Some people are certainly easier to hypnotise than others, but virtually anybody can be hypnotised very effectively by a hypnotherapist who knows what he or she is doing, and this can be done either in person or via a CD or DVD.

Myth 3: it's all mumbo-jumbo

People often think, *Well, there's no scientific proof to show that hypnosis works, so why should I believe it? It can't possibly work; after all, it's just some stranger telling you to behave in a certain way. Why would I take any notice of that?*

Fact It is certainly true that science has yet to come up with a definitive and watertight explanation for exactly how hypnosis works. But then, there is a lot that science does not yet understand about the workings of the human mind. Essentially, it is clear that when you are under hypnosis you are in a more 'suggestible' state. Scientific studies using electroencephalographs have found that under hypnosis the activity of the brain changes – it begins to show more sleep-like patterns than conscious, waking ones and also resistance is gone. And yet you feel lucid. In other words, it seems that during hypnosis the conscious mind – with all its doubts, fears and anxieties – takes a back seat. This allows the subconscious mind to open up.

> I will access your subconscious mind to help you to change your attitude to whatever you are addicted to.

The subconscious mind is responsible not just for your impulses and emotions but for your creativity and imagination too. As your hypnotherapist, I will delete unhelpful 'files' from your subconscious and replace them with helpful ones that you will then act upon, even when your conscious mind takes over.

Myth 4: hypnosis doesn't work

Some people find it difficult to believe that a person can change their behaviour, or cope with pain, simply by relaxing and listening while someone speaks to them in a quiet and peaceful way, and they feel certain that hypnosis couldn't possibly work for them.

Fact In over 23 years as a hypnotherapist I have seen countless people conquer their addiction problems using hypnotherapy. Women use hypnosis techniques to cope with the pain and anxiety of childbirth. People also use hypnosis to cope when undergoing dental work or to tackle long-held phobias.

But you don't have to take my word for this. There are numerous well-documented cases of hypnosis being used as the only form of anaesthesia for surgery, including gall-bladder removal, amputation, Caesarean section and hysterectomy. Hypnosis is used in medical settings around the world to help people cope with anything from cancer to allergies, gastrointestinal problems, chronic pain, burns, arthritis and hypertension (high blood pressure). It is also, of course, a well-established tool in mainstream psychotherapy, helping people to tackle issues such as anxiety or sleep disorders.

HYPNOQUIT tip
Background noise

It is always best to do your meditations when you are unlikely to be disturbed. Switch off your phones and shut the door. But this is the real world too, so you may hear noises coming from another room or outside while you are listening to the CD. These will not disturb you. It is normal to be aware of your surroundings during hypnosis, as your mind is in a state of increased and heightened awareness. The difference is that you will feel incredibly relaxed and free from tension. Even with some background noise, you can still reach a state of peace and tranquillity. You can listen to your CD on the train or bus providing your journey is longer than 20 minutes.

From now on, by using your daily meditations, you are going to delete from your subconscious mind the emotional associations that caused your addiction at the outset. You will no longer feel compelled to continue the addictive behaviours.

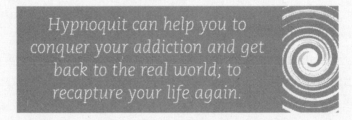

Hypnoquit can help you to conquer your addiction and get back to the real world; to recapture your life again.

You, and only you, know just how many times you have told yourself that this will be the last time. Hypnoquit will change all this. You can now reprogram your mind with a healthy approach to life – and to free yourself from this addiction for good! Chapter 15 explains everything you need to know to begin your first Hypnoquit session. The following chapters focus on different kinds of addiction. You may find that you actually have more than one, so it is worth reading through them all.

PART 2

UNDERSTANDING YOUR ADDICTION

5

IS EATING DOMINATING YOUR LIFE?

It may sound ridiculous to ask if you are a food addict. After all, we need food to survive and without it we would die. You wouldn't think that something that is life-sustaining, and which we all do, could be classed as addictive, would you? But I have seen thousands of people who are compulsively hooked on the very thing that is essential to life: food.

By the very nature of this subject, food is one of our biggest addictions worldwide, so this chapter is an important one for many people.

WHAT IS FOOD ADDICTION?

Recent studies have found that foods that are high in fat and sugar cause specific chemical changes in the brain, similar to the brain changes that happen when someone has used an opiate drug. This gives you that high – and it can be addictive, causing you to want more immediately. For many people it's sugary foods, white flour or refined carbohydrates that trigger this urge to binge. Chocolate is a favourite for many and gives the same high. Mints come a close second.

Food addiction can be overwhelming. When you start eating, the pleasure hits your brain and you just can't stop. You eat when you are not hungry. You eat food you don't particularly like the taste of, but if you are in the eating zone, food is food and it will do. You obsess about food – where, when and how you will eat next. You can't control your appetite because food is controlling you.

> Now you will learn quickly and easily how to plan meals, how to take control of the food you buy and the food you eat, and how to make healthy choices.

You may feel desperate, depressed, isolated, guilty and hopeless. You may feel like a failure. You may be slightly overweight or vastly overweight and full of self-loathing. Your self-esteem will have plummeted; in fact, you may be unable to remember what self-esteem is. You are almost certainly miserable.

What causes food addiction?

There can be any number of emotional reasons why people become addicted to food in this way. There may be past or present emotional trauma, stress or a seemingly well-intentioned and so-called 'helpful' comment from a loved one about your weight. Sometimes people become addicted to food as a response to traumatic events, such as bereavement, marital breakdown or redundancy.

Food addiction can be life threatening

Overeating can lead to obesity, causing many health problems, such as diabetes, heart disease, osteoarthritis, stroke, gallstones, infertility and depression, to name just a few. It can also lead to bulimia (bouts of extreme overeating followed by depression and self-induced vomiting), which can increase your risk of heart problems and do serious damage to your internal organs.

Furthermore, with bulimia, you may also experience hair loss and will most certainly damage your teeth because the contents of the stomach, which are vomited, contain acid. With females, menstruation stops.

So, anyone who tells you that food addiction somehow doesn't 'count' as a 'proper' addiction, or that it isn't 'serious', is wrong and they don't know what they are talking about. Food addiction can be just as dangerous and just as potentially life threatening as any addiction to drugs, cigarettes or alcohol. And it can make you just as desperate.

WHY DIETS ARE NOT THE ANSWER

Many of the food addicts I see are also diet addicts. Perhaps you recognise yourself here: you bounce from one regime to the other trying desperately to control your eating; your weight yo-yos and you become impatient for results; you ricochet between bingeing and starvation and become miserable, hungry and out of control. Yet you are still addicted, whatever the scales say at any given point, because the mind part hasn't been dealt with.

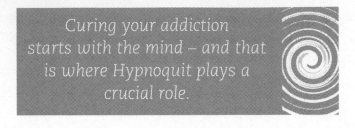

Curing your addiction starts with the mind – and that is where Hypnoquit plays a crucial role.

Diets fuel food addiction; they don't cure it

In all the years I have treated people for food addictions, I have seen time and time again how utterly pointless diets are. Diets only appear to work. Some diets are more effective than others in the short term, but they do not tackle the root cause of your food addiction, which is, quite simply, your mind.

I've heard many dieting horror stories over the years and have treated people who have spent their life savings on gastric bands, stomach stapling and liposuction – sometimes with life-threatening consequences.

★ **Case Study:** Caroline, 47 and a mother of three young boys, was so desperate to conquer her addiction to food that she turned to surgery.

Before treatment:

After having a gastric band fitted, Caroline suffered from complications. Her husband and mother were called to her bedside and the surgeon told them she probably wasn't going to make it. For a few horrendous hours, it looked like her boys were going to be left motherless. By a miracle, Caroline survived.

This is how bad food addiction can get. When she came to me, she was naturally still addicted to food, despite her operation and trauma, because the reason for her addiction hadn't been dealt with.

After treatment:
With Hypnoquit, Caroline was finally able to overcome the addiction. After just three sessions she told me she felt that at last she was in control.

Caroline's case seems extreme, but you'd be surprised how common these or similar experiences are. Most people who take desperate measures such as gastric bands do not conquer their addiction to food. One client, Harriet, a tax solicitor in her fifties, told me that in the weeks after her stomach stapling operation, because she could only eat puréed food and her craving for chocolate was so desperate, she would put Mars Bars in the blender. Other people tell me that they chew the food and when they have had enough taste and 'pleasure', they spit it out.

I hear more and more stories like this, and I feel their emotion, their utter desperation and pain, as more and more diets flood the market. But I'll say it loud and clear: diets don't work long term for most people. They are OK while you are on the diet and being monitored and restricted, but you cannot sustain a diet long term. When you come off the diet most people, in my experience of treating weight-loss clients, put all the weight back on and some more besides. Some diets work well and people manage to maintain their weight loss, but usually at a cost of never seeming to be able to relax and have a normal healthy relationship with food. I am assuming, since you are reading this chapter, that you are in the former category rather than the latter.

In my experience, dieting will only fuel your food addiction. More and more professionals are agreeing with what I've been advocating for over 23 years. Diets make you feel guilty or panicky about eating. They often drive you to eat more, not less, out of rebellion, despair and self-hatred, or for comfort. It's interesting, don't you think, that you eat 'for comfort' although it gives you no comfort at all – only fear and guilt.

> Hypnoquit is simple: it allows you to make peace with food, with your mind and with your body – for ever.

WHY MY APPROACH IS DIFFERENT

You may be reluctant to start this programme, thinking that I am taking away the very thing that gives you comfort: food. But I am not doing that at all. In fact, it's diets that do that, and where have they got you? I am going to help you to have a normal healthy relationship with food. You will be able to have treats and not be afraid; rather, you will rejoice and learn to think, *I can have chocolate and cheese, and still lose weight.* You can, of course, but you will only want these treats in moderation, otherwise you will not lose weight. You will find yourself doing this naturally. Diets mean deprivation; deprivation causes more problems and solves none.

If you are a food addict, gimmicky diets and detox regimes will not help you to develop a healthy relationship with food. They will simply worsen your addiction, making your behaviour around food even less normal.

Here's the truth: the only way to lose weight is to consistently consume fewer calories than you burn off (calories in versus calories out). You may do this for a short while on these diets – they all rely on getting you to eat fewer calories, whatever they say – but at what cost? Deprivation, low self-esteem and so on, just to labour the point.

With Hypnoquit, you will no longer feel anxiety and self-doubt about eating. As you do your daily meditations, you will replace your food cravings and self-criticism with self-acceptance and a wholesome relationship with food. Your self-esteem will skyrocket as you begin to see that you can lose your destructive addiction and eat normally.

Eat less, exercise more

We all know how to lose weight. It's no secret in that you must eat fewer calories than you expend (exercise) on a daily basis, but it is important to remember that for the body to be healthy this means having regular healthy meals and smaller portions and *not* skipping meals.

With the Hypnoquit programme you will want to do more to be healthy and trim, so exercise is an important part. Choose an exercise regime that you enjoy, and make it regular. Don't rush to join a gym (as gyms often scare people, especially if you have never been inside one), but start off by walking wherever you can every day. Also, use the stairs rather than the lift. If you enjoy swimming, make yourself a regular date once or twice a week at the local pool and swim a few lengths, increasing the number over the weeks. You'll feel great after any exercise.

HOW CAN HYPNOQUIT HELP?

Using the CD meditations, I'll teach you how to eat in a balanced, healthy way for the rest of your life. By accessing your subconscious mind – the part responsible for the urges and impulses – I will help you to break the triggers that cause your addiction. You will simply no longer give in to the impulse to graze or overeat. You will begin to eat smaller portions, to eat mindfully, and you will listen to your body at last.

You'll immediately see your behaviour change from 'I need food' to 'I'd like food but I don't need it, so I'll wait.' The impulse to snack may be there sometimes, but the connection between impulse and action is not made. You will develop a sense of calm and confidence.

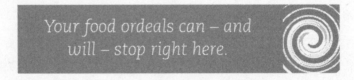

Your food ordeals can – and will – stop right here.

None of this is difficult or stressful. You'll learn to eat when you're hungry and stop when you have had enough to eat and you will enjoy the Hypnoquit process.

From now on, you are going to see food as pleasurable, life-sustaining nourishment, not an addiction. This may sound unlikely – impossible even – but believe me it works. I have seen so many people, just like you, liberate themselves from food addiction for ever.

I actually see most clients for only three sessions, and the results are amazing. Only recently someone texted me to say, 'I was weighed today and I wanted to let you know I have lost 4 stone!' Around 96 per cent of my clients take control of their eating habits easily and, as a result of this, achieve their goal size, lose weight and keep it off. They develop a normal, healthy relationship with food that is free of compulsion, guilt, control, diets or bingeing. The 4 per cent who struggle are simply not doing their self-visualisations. When they get a gentle but firm reminder from me, they are back on track again.

This method is not exclusive to people who see me in person. It's available to anyone, so you too can have the same results simply by listening to the CD and making your Visualisation Tool, which I will explain later in this chapter.

 ## HYPNOQUIT tip

Put away your bathroom scales

If you find this difficult to do now, don't worry, you will eventually realise you don't need them. Ideally, ditch the scales entirely, as they can be deceiving. While your waist is getting smaller in size, your actual weight could be going up due to several factors. Your body fluids fluctuate because you retain fluid sometimes, so your weight naturally fluctuates too. If you are exercising, the muscles you build up weigh more than the fat you're losing.

Weighing yourself will have fuelled your addiction in the past by making you unhappy, or making you feel you have 'failed'. You will have turned to the substance you craved: food. Not any more.

You'll know this method is working by how you feel about food – and you'll see the results of this by how your clothes fit. Throwing out the scales will seriously boost your 'feel-good factor'. This, in turn, will help to motivate you to keep up your daily meditations. No pressure though – throw away your scales in your own time.

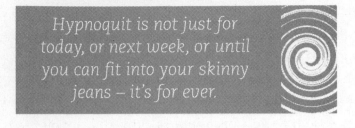

Hypnoquit is not just for today, or next week, or until you can fit into your skinny jeans – it's for ever.

In reality, this programme is not a regime at all. I won't be telling you about forbidden foods or have you counting calories, or insist you must go to the gym. This programme is about as enjoyable and laid back as you can get without jeopardising results.

WHAT IS A NORMAL HEALTHY RELATIONSHIP WITH FOOD?

Most food addicts I see have lost touch with what it is to eat normally. Many have abused food for so long that they can no longer hear what their body is telling them. 'I eat massive portions,' one client recently told me, 'but I never, ever feel full.'

A normal relationship with food is one that is free from guilt, self-punishment and emotional triggers. When you eat normally, you savour your food. You really enjoy eating, but you are not obsessed. You are in touch with your body. You choose foods that your body needs to stay healthy and fit for life. You might sometimes really want some chocolate or a piece of cheese. That's fine. But equally, sometimes you might really want blueberries or steamed broccoli.

My philosophy for normal eating is: everything in moderation. The 'moderation' part has been a major problem for you, but that was in the past. Moderation and healthy eating are the cornerstones of my approach. Any good nutritionist will tell you that this is the way to eat for life. And it is now the way *you* will eat for life.

The crucial thing is that from now on you will know what your body wants and needs – you will be in touch with yourself, not overcome by the mindless, powerful cravings that have ruled you for so long.

 HYPNOQUIT tip

Mindful eating

I am going to teach you, using the CD meditations, to savour your food, by eating slowly and becoming truly aware of what, and how, you are eating *while* you are eating. You will lose the panicky feelings associated with food, and replace them with calm ones. I call this eating mindfully and it means giving eating your full attention. This way you will enjoy your food, you won't rush through meals or feel driven to eat more and more. You will eat calmly and you will find it easy to stop when you have that 'had enough' feeling.

So, how do you do it? Well, it's incredibly simple. Although it may require some planning, and it will probably mean breaking some long-held bad habits, but you will enjoy it.

HOW TO EAT MINDFULLY

1 **Give eating your full attention.** Switch off the TV, the radio; put aside that newspaper or book. Sit down at a table and give your full attention to your meal.
2 **Appreciate your food:** arrange your food attractively on your plate and not haphazardly piled high in a mess. Take

in the colours, textures and the aromas before you eat – enjoy how amazing food can be.

3 **Really taste your food:** when you put the food into your mouth appreciate the tastes and textures on your tongue; enjoy the different flavours. This makes each bite a choice rather than a reflex or a habit. Excite your taste buds.

4 **Eat your favourite first.** Then if you leave food on your plate it doesn't matter, whereas if you leave your favourite until last, you will most likely eat too much. Also, the food tastes much better when you are hungry, so it stands to reason that the flavours of the favourite food will be even more pleasurable.

5 **Chew your food** – chew each mouthful 10 or 12 times. It's astonishing how fast most people eat. When you slow down, and chew and savour your food, you can tune into your body. When your brain sends the signal that you've had enough, you will listen. If you enjoy food so much why would you want to rush it? Extend the pleasure.

6 **Think about how you feel as you eat.** Ask yourself if you like the taste of the food you're choosing right now? How do you feel? Happy? Excited? Indifferent? Try not to judge the feeling. Simply observe it happening to you. Be curious about how eating makes you feel.

★ **Case Study:** Mary, 28, first came to see me when she was a size 18 and wanted to be a size 10.

Before treatment:

Mary had polycystic ovaries when she was 19, and had steadily gained weight since her diagnosis. Mary had tried every fad diet going. She was convinced each time that she would lose the weight and reach her goal, then stay on a controlled diet and never have to diet again. The next diet was always going to be *the* one, the *miracle*. This never happened. Mary had virtually given up when she met up with a friend who had lost over 12.7kg (2st/28lb) with Hypnoquit.

Mary was frustrated and tired of people who would say, 'It's a shame [about your weight], because you've got such a pretty face.' Even her dad would say, 'You'll be a stunner when you lose weight.' Mary had no boyfriend. She told me: *'I cry in private now and again. I don't think guys like me, as I am too fat. I hate shopping, and one day I said to my mum, "When I have lost some weight can we go shopping?" and she said, "No, and I am ashamed of you, your weight, the state of you – you've become very loud and aggressive too."*

'I was angry with her, but it's true: I have become aggressive and I obsess about eating, and I feel like a failure if I don't lose weight. I was size 8 up to 18 years of age then it all went wrong.

'I also have an addiction to mints and I buy them by the box. I can get through 8 packets just driving home from work and that's only 10 minutes away.

'I know that the shops around where I work and live are aware of my addiction and they are probably thinking, Here she comes again, but I don't care; I think, Just give me my mints and let me go. I have gum disease and I am too ashamed to tell my dentist about my addiction. If I don't get my mints I get jittery, and if I have cleaned the local shops out before their next delivery, I have been known to drive for miles to find some. I eat a certain brand and can't have any other brand at all. I never suck on them I chomp them. When I have had a binge, I don't eat all day and just slump in a chair and fall asleep.'

After treatment:

'Since I started Hypnoquit, I can visualise myself a size 10. All day, every day and I feel like singing and dancing, and I have an incredible amount of energy. I am so happy, because I can see changes in every area, some quite profound and some subtle. I haven't even thought about having a mint, which to me is amazing. I really can't believe it.

'I visualise myself wearing all the lovely clothes in my wardrobe. I never actually gave up on that – I always hoped I would be able to wear them again one day. I've also found that I love exercising too, and I must admit that I never, ever thought that would happen, never.

'I know it's a cliché to say this, but I just know this is the start of the rest of my life, a new me – a slim me.'

Mary took just six months to achieve her dream size 10, and had maintained this when I saw her again over one year later. Her mints were a distant memory. She was amused when I asked about her mints and couldn't quite believe that she had an addiction to them.

WHAT IS HEALTHY EATING IN PRACTICE?

Although I'm not promoting a diet as such, it helps to have an idea of portion sizes and healthy eating choices. Here are some guidelines:

Light meals

Here are some suggestions for tasty lunches or light main meals that will be nutritious and enjoyable.

- Stir-fry baby sweetcorn, cherry tomatoes and asparagus, plus lean protein of your choice – prawns, strips of chicken or beef, or cubes of tofu – then serve with blueberries sprinkled over the top.
- Salads: add fruit, such as mango, blueberries or strawberries, to your salads for a pleasant and refreshing change.
- Pan fry, in a little walnut oil, a salmon fillet (or other fish) coated in crushed walnuts for a tasty meal with health-giving omega-3s (see page 80). Serve with a few new potatoes and salad.
- Toast rye bread, spread thinly with almond or peanut butter and top with segments of clementines, satsumas or oranges.
- Make open sandwiches – they have less bread and look more appealing. (1) Try a mixture of thinly sliced chicken breast, avocado and freshly squeezed lime juice and top with salad leaves; (2) use slithers of cheese with sliced avocado, red onions, rocket and tomatoes; (3) mix avocado with lime or lemon juice and serve topped with smoked salmon.

Fruit and vegetables

A healthy diet includes plenty of fresh fruit and vegetables, preferably organic, to give you all the benefits of the vitamins and minerals contained in them. They also provide roughage, which is essential for feeling good and keeping your weight under control.

 HYPNOQUIT tip

Bright and healthy

Think of the spectrum of colours going from light colours to dark when you choose fruit and vegetables, and always have a preference for bright and dark, as they have an abundance of anti-carcinogenic

antioxidants, vitamins, minerals and fibre. All fruit and vegetables
have nutrients in them, of course, but bright and dark have more.

Go for as wide a selection of fruits and vegetables as you
can. Here are some suggestions:

- Enjoy red grapes, papaya, kiwi and peaches, as well as red
  peppers, tomatoes and beetroot.
- All berries – such as cherries, blueberries, blackberries and
  strawberries – are known as the 'super foods' and a must to eat
  daily. Goji berries, in particular, are little powerhouses. This
  super-antioxidant, high-protein berry from Asia is allegedly
  one of the highest antioxidant foods on earth.
- Eat health-giving fresh green leafy salads at least once a day
  and eat plenty of the leafy greens such as broccoli, Brussels
  sprouts, spinach and pak choi.
- Choose raw vegetables or fruit (especially berries) if you
  want a snack.
- In the winter, enjoy healthy home-made soups, preferably
  puréed, as you will feel fuller for longer.

Research shows that eating your five a day will not only slow
down the ageing process but will also significantly reduce your
risk of cancer and heart disease, as well as many other serious
conditions.

The energy-plus fruit

Bananas have excellent health benefits. I always have one
small banana a day and advocate you do too. There are
many misconceptions surrounding this invaluable fruit, usually

that they are considered 'too fattening', because they have a high sugar content. It is true that they contain sugars – three natural types of sugars: glucose, fructose and sucrose – but the body needs some natural sugars. Bananas give an instant energy boost and for this reason are favoured by athletes.

There is more to this fruit than just fitness benefits. Bananas are high in potassium, and they contain fibre, vitamin B6, all eight of the amino acids essential for health plus magnesium, iron and calcium. They help to lower cholesterol levels, and to treat depression and constipation. The abundance of potassium in bananas also helps your brain to stay alert, boosting your brainpower. In one study of 200 students made at Twickenham, Middlesex, those students who ate a banana for breakfast, break and lunch were more alert and achieved better exam results than those who did not eat bananas.

HYPNOQUIT tip
Eat fresh produce and live longer

Here is another good reason to make healthy choices. A recent television programme aimed to discover the secret of centenarians (people who are 100 years or older), and travelled to several places where there are higher percentages of these people. Two of the places studied were Okinawa and Sardinia. The Okinawans never over-ate and their diet comprised fish, fruit and lots of vegetables, but no meat, whereas the Sardinians ate a similar diet of fresh produce as well as suckling pigs. The important point here is that there were no prepared foods such as sugars, pasta, cakes, biscuits, chocolate or dairy produce in their diets. These people were happy, healthy, fit and active with sharp minds.

Fish oils benefit your health – BIG time

Eating omega-3 oils, found abundantly in oily fish, is the key to heart, brain and joint health and to a longer, healthier life. Omega-3 significantly reduces your risk of heart disease and stroke, because it maintains optimum blood pressure and cholesterol levels. It improves brain development and memory function, and is referred to as the perfect brain food. It also reduces your risk of certain cancers, diabetes and arthritis, and research has proven that it also helps to reduce depression and mood swings. Furthermore, omega-3 also gives you healthier and younger-looking skin (because it improves its elasticity), plus thick, healthy and shiny hair, and more flexible joints.

Food sources of omega-3 enter the bloodstream quickly and are therefore preferable to taking supplements, but you need to eat oily fish three times a week to get sufficient levels. Because these oils are so beneficial, however, this is one supplement I would highly recommend you take. Look for good-quality cold-pressed omega-3 oil that is mercury-free (certain oily fish, such as tuna, contain some mercury, which is removed in the better-quality supplements) and take one 1,000mg capsule daily.

Foods rich in omega-3 include herrings, salmon, mackerel, sardines, anchovies and scallops. Other sources include walnuts, walnut oil, flax seeds, flax seed oil, cabbage, pumpkin seeds, soya beans and romaine lettuce, although there are lower levels in these foods.

Although tuna and swordfish have an abundance of omega-3 they also contain mercury, so health experts recommend eating those fish no more than twice a week.

KEEPING A FOOD DIARY

A good way to help you to unpick the emotional associations that cause your food addiction is to keep a food diary. This will help you to understand your triggers: the feelings or events that drive you to food time and time again when you are not hungry. All you need is a small notebook that you can carry with you at all times. You will quickly see each day's improvements, and then after a while you will no longer need to keep the diary going.

How it's done

Use two pages for each day:

Page 1 note down what you eat and drink, and the times, throughout the day. This shows how regular your eating patterns are, how early you start eating and how late you finish. Are you a 'grazer' (you eat constantly throughout the day) or do you tend to skip meals? Do you have evening binges?

Page 2 note down your daily exercise and the length of time. Also note your general emotions throughout the day: if something or someone annoys you, for example, or makes you feel happy. You will begin to see patterns emerging and a correlation with food and emotions. Note down if you feel tired for no apparent reason or have a bloated stomach. This can indicate food intolerances. It is possible to develop a food intolerance seemingly quite out of the blue, and it can go as quickly as it came.

Keeping a food diary in this way will help you to build up a clearer picture of your addiction – what you eat, when and why; what drives you again and again to eat when you don't need it. Sometimes, it's only when we see it in black and white that we begin to understand not just what triggers our food addiction, but also what encourages us to eat healthily. In simple terms, how the addiction works.

 HYPNOQUIT tip

Keep it small

Make the diary small and light so that it will fit into your pocket or slot into your handbag.

★ **Case Study:** Karen, 33, is single and a City trader. At a size 18 she very much wanted to be a size 12.

Before treatment:

'I have hormone issues and I don't eat for two days sometimes and then I just pig out. If people see me eating I always feel guilty so I have to eat in secret.

'I actually like the full feeling in my stomach – that stuffed, can't-eat-anymore feeling – but I don't want to be like that anymore. I know it's no good for me and I will never lose weight eating so much food. I know all these things, sbut yet I don't do them.

'I never eat breakfast, and although I know it's just a case of training myself to eat it I find that difficult. I eat the usual junk: chocolate, crisps, cakes, biscuits, pasta and cheese. I stuff my face with food. It's all stodgy, starchy and sugary – I just love carbs and I can't seem to get enough of them. And I drink lots of diet soda.

'I kid myself that if I just don't eat I will lose weight, so I am really happy if I can go a long time without eating, but I'm a size 18 so how can this be a fact? I still kid myself, though.

'Occasionally, I go out with my friends, but I eat small amounts. Then I start punishing myself with my thoughts like, They are probably thinking how come she's so fat if we hardly see her eating, and when she does it's not much. I stopped drinking alcohol for a while because I read that it's just empty calories. I thought that would help, but it didn't.

'Also I never exercise. I am a mess and I want to change. My sisters are both a size 8, so I feel even fatter when we have to get together for family occasions.'

After treatment:
'After the first session, I haven't been snacking at all, which is a miracle. I feel that it is a natural process and it seems to take all the drama out of losing weight. It has been incredibly easy, I must admit. I had a problem seeing myself slim in my visualisation, but I can do that now and it makes a big difference.'

Karen worked with Hypnoquit and achieved her goal size of a small size 12 within four months. She has a boyfriend and says this is the happiest time of her life right now. She had a few minor setbacks along the way, but with a gentle but firm reminder from me, to practise her 20 minutes' visualisation every day, she soon got back on track. Karen believed it would work for her, and it did.

CREATE A PICTURE OF THE NEW, SLIM YOU AS YOUR VISUALISATION TOOL

Although this may sound rather strange, creating a Visualisation Tool – a picture of your addiction-free self – really does help to reinforce your efforts to eat sensibly and healthily.

In Chapter 15, when I explain all about making such a picture, I want you to visualise yourself the size you really *want* to be, even though your hopes of achieving this have probably been dashed many times in the past. You will probably decide to imagine a size that you think is more realistic, but I say, don't go for that 'realistic' size, be bold and go for your *dream size* – and don't be afraid to do so!

You may have a favourite photograph of yourself taken when you were the ideal size, or you may prefer to flip through a magazine to find an image of the perfect body size – a size you've dreamed of becoming and you know this will be your body shape. Superimpose your face from a favourite photograph onto the image of that ideal body. If you're a computer whiz, you may have a better way of doing this that allows you to print out a more 'realistic' picture of your own face on this ideal body. Now turn to pages 214–16 to learn how to finish making your Visualisation Tool and how to use it.

> *Your dream size can become a reality.*

HOW HYPNOQUIT WILL HELP YOU TO CONQUER YOUR FOOD ADDICTION

It's simple, and it can start right now. From your very first session listening to the CD, doing your daily meditation, your visualisations and affirmations, you will lose the craving and obsession for food. You will find yourself drawn to healthier eating. You will stop eating when you've reached that 'had enough to eat' feeling. You will reduce – or even eliminate – the impulse to snack. You will also begin to see food as an enjoyable fuel for your body.

What is more, you will see what a positive part of your life exercise can be and begin to see exercise as an essential part of your daily life and not an optional extra.

 HYPNOQUIT tip

Rearrange your fridge contents

Put the 'naughty' food, such as chocolate and cheese, in the vegetable drawer – hidden – and put the vegetables on the shelves so that you can see them as soon as you open the fridge door. Luxuriate in all those bright colours. When you are in an unhealthy eating zone it's the 'naughty' food you are looking for, but this will soon change to looking at the healthy zone.

In my experience you will have been constantly opening the fridge door and just looking into it. You may close it sometimes without eating, but you will certainly be looking in there several times during the day. These moments will get fewer as each day progresses after starting the Hypnoquit programme, until finally you will look into the fridge only when you are preparing a meal or when you are hungry; however, it removes any temptation if you are met with an array of vegetables and not cake, chocolate or cheese. This really does work and I have all my clients doing this effectively.

★ **Case Study:** Martina, 44, was addicted to chocolate.
Before treatment:
Martina was 71kg (11st 3lb/157lb) when she started the programme and lost 2.7kg (6lb) in the first week. The next week, she steadily lost another 1.3kg (3lb). Thanks to her meditations and visualisations, she had also lost the obsession with chocolate that had been ruling her since having children.

'My addiction to chocolate got steadily worse over the years. It got so bad that I'd eat chocolate instead of meals. I'd have five toffee crisps, four Kit Kats, a huge bar of chocolate and a full packet of chocolate biscuits in one sitting. My husband would have a meal, but I didn't want any at all, I preferred chocolate. Of course, I would always say I had eaten, I wouldn't want my husband or anyone to know about my addiction.

After treatment:
'There are a lot of heart problems and diabetes in my family, and as I am overweight I know I need to watch what I eat more than most people. I must admit I was sceptical about Hypnoquit, but it's been so much easier than I thought it could possibly be and it has been enjoyable.

'I haven't really done diets. I used to run in the park and eat very healthily until I had my children, then it all seemed like too much trouble. If someone asked if I wanted vegetables I always said no, but since I have been hypnotised, I want to eat healthily. Also, I love seeing myself slim in the visualisations –

it really works so well. It makes the whole process enjoyable and very easy.

'I used to eat chocolate in the car, in secret, anywhere I could get hold of some, but now I don't crave it any more. I have berries or raw carrots instead if I feel peckish. And I drink lots of water. Yesterday was a real test for me: I was in my "chocolate shop" but I bought just a single chocolate, instead of all the chocolate bars I used to get, and I haven't eaten it yet.

'The other day at work there were cakes and biscuits, but I didn't have any. I realised I just didn't fancy any. I keep thinking of my visual image. I am so thrilled. This is a revelation for me.

'I had the smallest bag of chocolates possible at the cinema and I ate a few and then gave them to my children. That's unheard of for me. Whether I am at work, or at home, or out and about, I know I will be fine. I have proved it to myself.

'I am very sensitive, so I have to remember that if anyone has a problem with me, it's their problem and not mine, so I will no longer have a need to eat for comfort. I want to be really assertive and not a pushover, and I feel that Hypnoquit is already helping me to do that too.

'I absolutely love doing the self-hypnosis. I enjoy the peace and quiet of it. My friends think I have become like a woman possessed, and they laugh, but I am ecstatic. Interestingly, two of my friends are intrigued and are talking about doing Hypnoquit themselves.'

Hypnoquit works by reprogramming your mind. No gimmicks. No fads.

So there you have it. You are going to reprogram your mind from the inside out, so that the link between emotions, cravings, obsessions and food is broken – for good. You will feel so free when you lose this addiction, you will see results straight away and become the person you always knew you could be.

Read Part 3, then use the action plan in Chapter 16 to help you get started.

6

IS SHOPPING AN OBSESSION THAT YOU CAN'T CONTROL?

Do you get a high from shopping, a feeling of elation or excitement when you make that purchase? Do you max out your credit cards, feel euphoric for a while, and then quickly feel guilty and depressed about what you've done – again? Do you hide your purchases? Do you take desperate measures – deceit, borrowing money and concealing your credit-card bills – to cover up your shopping habits? Are you in debt, but do you still shop nevertheless? If any of this rings true, then you are most likely a shopping addict.

Do you shop madly, get the high, then return everything – and get another high from doing so? I call this 'reverse shopping' and you don't have to be an addict to do this. In my experience of treating shopping addictions, many of my clients think that buying loads of goodies one week and then taking them all back the next week is an addiction and not normal behaviour. It can be an addiction, this is true to say, although it can also mean someone who is indecisive, who buys clothes, shoes, bags and so on, in the glamour of the stores and with encouragement from the charming shop assistant, who then simply changes their mind when they get home. They then take them back the following week, or they will hang on to them for a while just in case they change their mind again. This person is not an addict, just indecisive.

I have treated thousands of shopping addicts over the years and, interestingly, some don't always recognise their addiction, or they are in denial. Sometimes during treatment for something completely different, they ask for help with their shopping, which has 'got out of control', when they discover that it is in fact an addiction.

The unbearable need to buy

Shopping addiction – 'oniomania' is the technical term for it – is the compulsive urge to buy things. It is also known as compulsive shopping, compulsive buying or shopaholism, and it is a growing problem in our society. One recent study found that around 9 per cent of the American population are shopping addicts.

WHEN YOU BUY FOR THE HIGH

Shopping addicts invariably get more enjoyment from buying the goodies than they do out of wearing or using them. Often, their cupboards will be full of new purchases: shoes and racks of clothes with the price tags still attached. It's not unusual for a shopping addict, when having a clear out or looking for that old favourite pair of shoes, to come across items that are still in the bag, hidden at the back of the closet from family members. New shoes may get a single outing, but clothes are often never worn at all.

Shopaholics will go shopping with the intention of buying one or two items, but often come back laden with several bags. In some cases they can have emotional amnesia; they simply don't remember buying the items, which is quite extraordinary when you think about it. Many of my shopaholic clients have exclaimed, 'Where did that come from? I don't remember buying that!' when they come across it much later, in the back of the closet.

Shopping addiction is not exclusive to the rich and famous who are seemingly able to afford it. In fact, income doesn't come into the equation at all, as you will see from the extreme examples in this chapter. Shopaholics are often in denial about their addiction, even when they cannot pay their household bills and their credit rating is suffering. When this happens, they may simply take all the clothes and items back for a refund the following week (reverse shopping) and start the process all over again.

The effects of this behaviour can be devastating, as I'm sure you know all too well if you are addicted. An addiction to shopping can take over your entire life, causing financial and emotional turmoil.

★ **Case Study:** Charlotte, 35, and recently married, was addicted to shopping.
Before treatment:
One January she took herself off to New York for a post-festive detox at a fabulous spa. Within half an hour of checking into her hotel, she found herself on Fifth Avenue, handing over her credit card for an $8,500 Hermes bag.

Meanwhile, back in London, the Amex company were calling her husband to suggest they were going to put a suspension on the card, suspecting fraud. However, this was not the first time her husband had got a call like this from other credit-card companies. He asked Amex to wait a couple of hours while he checked with his wife. When he finally reached her, he got the answer he suspected.

That Hermes bag would have been cheaper in London. But the thrill would not have been the same had Charlotte waited for a few days. She already had a closet full of designer bags, and credit-card bills amounting to thousands of pounds. She didn't even particularly like the colour of this newly acquired Hermes bag, but the desire, the impulse that was driving her to spend $8,500 right there and then on Fifth Avenue, was overpowering.

After treatment:

Charlotte realised through hypnosis that there were other things in life that could give her pleasure apart from shopping and that she had been neglecting her husband. She had previously always been too busy and impatient to listen to him because she was obsessed with having 'me' time and spending money. She realised that even though newly married, they were almost leading separate lives. All that changed through hypnosis, and within a matter of four weeks Charlotte was fully recovered and decided to retrain in marketing so that she could help her husband in his business. She felt as though her eyes had been opened for the first time about the qualities she and her husband brought to their relationship.

Questionnaire:
Are you a compulsive shopper?

	Yes	No
Do you often spend more than you can afford?	☐	☐
Do you shop when you are feeling unhappy, to try to change your mood?	☐	☐
Do you often buy things you don't need?	☐	☐
Do you shop for a 'quick fix' to make you feel empowered?	☐	☐
Do you feel guilty or ashamed after you have shopped?	☐	☐
Are many of your purchases hidden or unused?	☐	☐
Do you repeatedly buy the same items, such as shoes?	☐	☐
Have your attempts to stop been unsuccessful?	☐	☐

If you answered 'yes' to four or more of the above questions, you have a shopping problem.

Let Hypnoquit help you to break your cycle of compulsive shopping.

WHAT CAUSES SHOPPING ADDICTION?

Our emotions and shopping behaviour are inextricably linked. A shopping addiction, for instance, can be the result of boredom, anger, fear or loneliness. Many of my clients are experiencing stress in the home, at work, at college or school, or are in unhappy relationships. Many feel insecure or that they are not important as a person. Many have troubled backgrounds (shopaholism can have its roots in childhood unhappiness, for example).

Some of my clients tell me how neglected they felt because of their parents' busy lives when they were growing up, or how lonely and unloved they felt. They often have very low self-esteem as a result. Sometimes they talk about how 'things' (toys or belongings) were their main companions in childhood.

Many shopping addicts simply cannot cope with the emotions they are feeling (or burying). So they repress these feelings, temporarily, by buying things, as in childhood, for example.

Most of us have heard of the expression 'an addictive personality' and you may have been labelled, or indeed you may have labelled yourself, as such.

OUR 'GIVE ME MORE' SOCIETY

It doesn't help that today's society is constantly pushing more and more tempting merchandise at us. Consumerism is rife in the modern world. Everywhere you look there are adverts persuading you that you 'need' more than you already have or that you'll feel complete if you buy this bag or that desirable dress, the latest must-have miracle face cream, or that scrumptious trendy sofa. What's more, it is now possible to get a full set of credit cards to fund even the most chronic, compulsive shopping behaviour. Our consumer society enables and fuels shopping addiction.

Internet shopping has also become popular these days, and many people develop a shopping addiction this way. According to the Office for National Statistics in the UK, just 3.9 per cent of retail sales take place online. But even so, that still represents millions of pounds in money spent.

Shopping statistics

According to figures published by the Centre for Retail Research in February 2010:

- UK shoppers spent about £38 billion shopping online in 2009.
- This amount is still only about 10 per cent of the total shopping in the UK.
- It is predicted that UK shoppers will spend over £42 billion in 2010.
- The average amount spent by individual shoppers in 2009 (who shopped online) was £1,102.
- UK shoppers spent more online than anywhere else in Europe in 2009, accounting for almost one-third of all European sales.

HOW DOES A SHOPPING ADDICTION TAKE HOLD?

For a few moments, while you are planning and making your purchases, you feel excited, satisfied and happy – even elated. For a short while, your stresses or troubles seem to have vanished into thin air. You feel alive, ecstatic and free. But this so-called 'retail therapy' is not therapy at all. In fact, it is downright destructive.

You walk around town (well, almost skip), happily swinging your bags. You may meet friends for coffee to show off your latest purchases. Or you may be very secretive.

Almost as soon as you get home these positive feelings vanish. They are replaced by guilt, anxiety, self-hatred or blame. Often you have to hide your loot to avoid being berated for your spending.

Like all addictions, this is a downward spiral. To make yourself feel better, you reach for the credit card again. You buy more and more stuff, just to get that same happy rush. Your home is filling up with purchases you do not want, like or need. Your wardrobe and your cupboards are bursting with clothes, shoes, bags and objects that you'll never wear or use, and your finances may be under catastrophic strain.

You start to feel ashamed. Some of my clients even destroy, give away or throw out the things they have bought, because they cannot face them, or the thought that they might be discovered.

There are people who spend hours after their latest spree totting up everything they have spent with a growing sense of panic, whereas others are in denial and never check their bank statements at all. But as the reality of what they've done kicks in, so do the feelings of depression and worthlessness.

> *Your feelings of guilt, shame and anxiety will drift away as Hypnoquit guides you towards managing your shopping in a controlled way.*

★ **Case Study:** Mia, 43, would go shopping every day. Even if it was just for the latest mascara or sun top, she had to have something.
Before treatment:
Weekends were her favourite times, because she could indulge and spend the whole two days shopping. For her,

the high was topped up every time she bought something new, no matter how large or small. Any purchase would do. Her day was filled with immense thrill and excitement, and she was immune to the comments her boyfriend would make about her spending – until holiday time came around.

They had booked to go away in the summer, but when the time came to buy the tickets, Mia simply had no money. Her credit cards were up to max. So, no holiday! After much debate, her boyfriend paid for her to go on holiday on the condition that she would 'get it sorted'. So she did, with the Hypnoquit programme.

After treatment:

Mia realised that her boyfriend was more than disappointed with her and she feared losing him through what she called her 'mindless behaviour'. Her boyfriend now went shopping with her and she was able to shop for essential items only; however, with the help of Hypnoquit, Mia was confident that she would be able to do this whether he was there or not. She lost the interest in 'mindless' shopping.

HOW OTHERS SUFFER

Not surprisingly, shopping addiction can put a terrible strain on relationships. Addictions are very difficult for partners or loved ones to live with. They are affected by the behaviour but might find it hard to understand or to sympathise with. They may even, sometimes, be unable to recognise what is happening. Loved ones will be baffled, angry or bemused. What may have seemed cute at the start of a relationship soon becomes a problem.

HOW CAN HYPNOQUIT HELP YOU?

Put simply, Hypnoquit will enable you to quickly and effectively 'delete' the association in your mind between your emotions and needs and your credit card.

There is no need for you to go back over your childhood and unearth the painful causes of your shopping addiction, because the hypnosis does this for you.

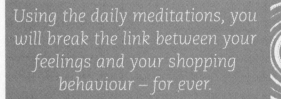

Using the daily meditations, you will break the link between your feelings and your shopping behaviour – for ever.

You may still feel upset or stressed at times. We all do, that's everyday life, but when you feel this way, thanks to your daily meditations, the impulse to translate them into a shopping spree will simply be gone. You will no longer feel drawn to shopping as the solution or escape route. You'll see the effects of this immediately.

Free at last!

Clients tell me how incredibly liberating it felt to lose that urge to shop. 'It was like being let out of a prison,' says Annabel, 33, a beauty therapist. 'I felt I could breathe again. Nothing was driving me or pulling at me or tormenting me. I was free, and in control.'

You will also, through your daily meditations, learn to boost your self-esteem and self-worth. This will help you to feel more confident and calm, less stressed or panicky. You will soon realise that you have so much to offer as a person, and that a life free from this addiction – and all the problems that come with it – is truly worth living to the full.

The guided meditations on the CD will encourage you to develop even more of your own affirmations and use them to change the way you feel. This, in turn, will liberate you from the urge to shop.

HYPNOQUIT tips

How to quit a shopping addiction for ever

- **Know your closet.** As you start the programme, take the time to organise your closet. Group your dresses together and your jackets and tops, and so on. Also, colour-code your clothes, grouping similar colours together within each category. When you have done this, you will see clearly how many clothes you actually have. You will discover hidden clothes too – all shopaholics have these. So, it's like shopping in your own closet and getting a whole new wardrobe!
- **Get support.** Tell a close friend or relative that your shopping has become uncontrollable, and you may want to tell them that you are helping yourself by doing Hypnoquit. Ask them to help you kick this addiction by supporting you and encouraging you.
- **Address the inner need.** When you get the urge to shop, write down what you are actually feeling. This will help you to think about the specific emotional needs you are trying to fulfil by shopping. When you have worked out what drives you to shop, try to think of other ways to fill that need; for example, if

you feel lonely in the daytime when your partner is at work and you are at home, sign up for voluntary work or arrange to meet up with friends.

- **Recognise the urge to shop.** If you keep a note of your emotions and what you are doing when you get the urge to shop, you will also be able to identify patterns. Do you get the urge to shop when bored? Or during your lunch hour, as stress relief? Or every evening on the way home as a 'pick me up'? Identifying patterns can help you to change your behaviour.
- **Spend within your budget.** Be aware of your weekly budget and make lists of the essential items, the comfort items and the luxury items. This will help and encourage you to exercise control over your spending, as you will be able to see where you can make cuts. You will begin to feel empowered. Think of the money you have saved by not shopping and see it building up in your bank account.

DON'T FOOL YOURSELF

You may think that your addiction to shopping is somehow containable. You may think, *Well, it's only shopping, it's not drugs or booze – and anyway everyone shops*, but not everyone has a shopping addiction. I've learned over the years from working with countless clients that a shopping addiction can ruin lives – and it tends to escalate. It really can spiral out of control.

> *Addictions become less pleasurable but more compulsive as the addiction advances.*

Now is the time to conquer your shopping behaviour for good. No more excuses – it is time to end this destructive addiction. The sense of freedom (not to mention the boost to your bank account) will feel amazing!

Read Part 3, then use the action plan in Chapter 16 to get started.

7

HAS YOUR DESIRE FOR SEX MADE YOU IRRESPONSIBLE, UNCARING AND RECKLESS?

Having sexual desires and enjoying sexual activity are as normal as breathing, for healthy men and women. But what happens when your sexual behaviour, your urges and sex drive, get out of control and lead to areas of your life being negatively affected? What happens when the physical act and thoughts of sex dominate your mind, making it difficult to conduct healthy personal relationships and interfering with your daily life?

The term 'sexual addiction' is used to describe the behaviour of a person who has an unusually intense sex drive or an obsession with sex and who is unable to control their sexual behaviour. It can cause professional and social problems for you and cause you to hurt the ones you love.

What are the signs of sexual addiction?

- If your sexual behaviour causes relationship, career, emotional or physical consequences, but you continue to engage in the same sexual behaviour, you do have a problem.
- If your sexual behaviour takes up more time and energy than you want to give it or if this behaviour causes you to continually behave in ways that go against your underlying values and beliefs, and yet you are unable to stop it, then you are probably a sex addict.

EXCESSIVE COMPULSION EQUALS ADDICTION

Sex addicts, both men and women, often say to themselves, 'This is the last time,' yet they feel compelled to indulge in the same sexual situations. It is scientifically determined that an excessive compulsion towards sex is one form of psychological addiction, just like smoking, substance abuse or alcoholism.

Addicts engage in various forms of sexual activity, despite the negative and dangerous consequences, damaging the addict's relationships and giving no thought to sexually trans-mitted diseases (STDs) and unwanted pregnancies; in fact, they often have an illusion that they are immune to both.

HOW DOES SEXUAL ADDICTION WORK?

As with most addictions, it is difficult to pinpoint the exact and main cause of a sexual addiction, and it could be the result of several conditions and circumstances. People who are sex addicts are often caring, sensitive, loving people who have become vulnerable to addictions because they have experienced an emotional trauma in either their first intense intimate relationship or friendship, or during childhood, and were not equipped with the tools to deal with it. They hate their behaviour and impulses; they despise themselves for behaving in this way, but they can't stop. They are out of control.

Sex addicts often deny that they have a problem. They make excuses for their actions, blaming others for what is happening, and they will do anything other than face up to the fact that their behaviour is out of control.

This distorted thinking provides an excellent distraction – for a while. If this is you, you may find yourself rationalising and justifying your behaviour, even when you know that it is wrong and harmful.

The buzz of the risk

Sex addiction is also bound up with risk taking. When you have obsessive sexual thoughts or encounters, you get a temporary high. This feeling has nothing to do with loving and caring for another person. It is reckless, selfish and unfeeling, but it is absolutely compelling. It takes you over. I have treated clients who have had unsafe sex with strangers in the bathroom of a restaurant, while their beloved spouse sits at the table, completely unaware.

Other common sex-addict behaviours include:

- Compulsive masturbation.
- Having multiple affairs and infidelities.
- Excessive use of pornography, online or otherwise.
- Becoming compelled by cybersex (virtual online sexual-fantasy encounters, discussed on page 109).
- Having unsafe or risky sex.

★ **Case Study:** Jack, 28, is a trainee accountant who came to see me about a sex addiction.

Before treatment:

'In many ways, I must have seemed like the ideal boyfriend. I am loving, attentive and solvent. Sam and I had lots of fun together, I made her laugh. I love to cook and clean, and she says I am handsome. But I failed her so badly, because of my behaviour.

'At first, our relationship was amazing. We had great sex and we knew how to make each other happy. She started to move her stuff into my flat. Maybe it was that that started it – a fear of commitment, who knows – but I began to have this secret life. I started having casual one-off sex with other women, usually picking them up in bars, during a night out with my mates. I somehow managed to think of this as something separate from my relationship with Sam. But we slowly stopped having sex. I began to have more and more of these sexual encounters instead. At one point I picked up a girl at Paddington station at 10.00 a.m. I was out of control.

'Weirdly, the rest of our relationship never changed. We loved each other and had fun together. But eventually I knew I couldn't go on like this. I broke down and confessed what I'd been doing. She understandably left me.

'I now think if I'd spoken to her right at the start about this compulsion, we'd still be together. If I'd got help earlier, she might have understood that it was an addiction. It was the secrecy and the high of the risk that kept me doing it, even with the dreadful guilt afterwards. I miss Sam so badly, but she's proud and she won't take my calls. I need to quit this behaviour for ever. If only I'd tried Hypnoquit earlier but, in a way, I didn't want to quit then. Now I do. I've lost the woman I love and I want to stop before it happens again and before I ruin my life.'

After treatment:

It's better to tell loved ones earlier rather than later. Jack is now in a loving relationship with someone who has a similar personality to his previous girlfriend Sam, and he has stopped his compulsion completely. He had a strong desire to succeed with beating his addiction, as he blamed this for losing Sam. He is now happy and moving on with his life. He realises that he has made mistakes but has learned to not dwell on the past.

SEX ADDICTS ARE NOT MONSTERS

If you are a sex addict, you probably gain little satisfaction from your encounters or activities, other than at the outset of your addiction. You'll invariably reject any emotional bond with your sexual partners. But you are not a monster – far from it. In fact, most of the people I have worked with tell me that their first experience of sex was fun, exciting, loving and bonding. They just can't understand how they have gone from this kind of experience to sexual encounters that are irresponsible, uncaring and reckless.

PORNOGRAPHY, INTERNET PORNOGRAPHY AND CYBERSEX

Addiction to pornography relates to the excessive use of pornographic material that interferes with daily life. It has its roots in video pornography and magazines, but these days, with the Internet in most homes and virtually every workplace, sex addicts often go online for a new and accessible way to satisfy their craving for sex.

Some people become addicted to virtual sex on the Internet, and some take this a step further and use the Internet to have anonymous sexual encounters for one-night stands. Others, however, are hooked on cybersex – virtual fantasy sexual encounters. By using a webcam, porn addicts can also indulge in online sex with strangers, and some pay for this service (online prostitution).

With sexual addiction, this behaviour goes way beyond curiosity or exploration. It becomes a time-consuming compulsion, overruling normal, healthy relationships and impulses. Someone with a porn addiction tends to isolate themselves, spending hours or even days in their own world of sexual fantasy, masturbation and guilt.

To ascertain whether your interest in pornography is an addiction, please answer the following questions on page 108.

Questionnaire:
Are you a pornography addict?

	Yes	No
Do you struggle to control your thoughts about pornography?	☐	☐
Does your pornography habit stop you from fulfilling other commitments to your family, friends or colleagues?	☐	☐
Do you use pornography to escape from other feelings?	☐	☐
Have you promised yourself that you'll quit/throw away your materials only to replace them/go online again?	☐	☐
Do you become distressed or angry if someone asks you to quit your addictive behaviour?	☐	☐
Do you attempt to hide your addiction and go to great lengths to keep it a secret?	☐	☐

If you answered 'yes' to four or more, you have an addiction.

> *Hypnoquit has helped many people leave their sex addiction behind and make a fresh start.*

A pornography addiction can slowly become your daily life – taking up more and more of your time, energy, and thoughts. You may take huge risks in order to satisfy your craving for pornography.

The hold of Internet porn

Internet pornography is highly addictive because it is:

- **Easy to access.** Around 28,000 Internet users are viewing pornography every second of the day.
- **Explicit.** It is possible to find material to satisfy any urge or taste.
- **Private.** You can do it without anyone ever knowing.

You discover more and more intense highs as you surf the Internet for new or increasingly hardcore material – fuelling your addiction as you seek that ever more elusive 'buzz'.

ESCAPISM AND PORNOGRAPHY

You may spend hours and hours in the privacy of your home, engaging in fantasies that are completely impossible in real life. This is addictive escapism. Not surprisingly, many of my clients also tell me that their Internet pornography and/or cybersex addiction has replaced genuine intimate relationships.

With cybersex – a virtual sex encounter – you enter a kind of fantasy world where participants describe their own actions, evoking graphic mental images in each other's minds. More confident participants might use webcams to share images as well as words. This form of role playing can become highly addictive – it is an escape from the real world, just like taking drugs, or drinking alcohol, except this high is fuelled by the mind. It is a break from the harsh reality of daily life.

A 31-year-old man I treated some time ago would have webcam sex early in the morning before going to work and occasionally he'd even go home at lunchtime when the urge was too powerful for him to control. Masturbation in the toilets at work wasn't enough for him.

If you're using a virtual world, such as Second Life, the anonymity of going online allows you to become someone different. It is an escape, but also a form of self-expression. You can become whatever you want to be online – younger, single, thinner. You can change the colour of your hair, your body shape – everything about yourself. Under this cloak of anonymity, you can also explore things you would never allow yourself to express in 'real' life. This can escalate. And as it does, the need for secrecy – the shame and guilt – grows too.

Like any addiction, pornography, Internet pornography or cybersex addiction can destroy relationships and careers. Before you know it, your life has become that computer screen. There is often nothing else. By day you work; by night you chase the sexual high – on a computer.

WHAT HAPPENS WHEN YOU QUIT?

When you make the brave decision to quit your addiction, you may feel shame, embarrassment and sometimes humiliation. You may also have to contend with some serious relationship issues. This is assuming your partner knows about your addiction, or you decide to tell them. You may not have been aware, while you were in the depths of your addiction, that your partner has been suffering, feeling neglected and alone. Your partner will feel hurt, betrayed, jealous and angry. Partners of sex or pornography addicts tend to compare their bodies to the images online, which the addict is viewing. Their self-esteem plummets, as they assume that their partner prefers that body type to theirs.

As with all addictions, the decision to quit has to come from you, and you alone. In many cases, it takes a significant event such as a relationship crisis to force the addict to admit to their problem and to get help. This always happens later than their partner or spouse would like it to, but at least they have made that first step at last.

> *Have you now reached the decision that you are going to quit?*

★ **Case Study:** Mary is married to Jim, who was an online pornography addict for 17 years.

Before treatment:

When she brought her husband to see me, she was angry and hurt. She talked openly about how his online porn addiction had affected her.

'I actually resent my computer for being available for Jim to view girls, to fantasise and masturbate. He never wants to have sex with me and always says he's too tired. I go to bed before him but I know what he's doing. I feel so betrayed and jealous, angry and hurt. It feels like another woman is in our life competing for his attention. This addiction is cruel. Because of it, Jim shows no regard for my feelings at all. Even though I am not an addict myself, I need help to deal with my self-esteem and anger now. I've brought Jim to have the treatment with me because he is ready to quit – he says he is – but I need help too.'

Jim was very quiet while Mary talked. He nodded from time to time. He knew how devastating his behaviour had become, and how out of control. He then told me he desperately wanted to stop; he could see that he was hurting his wife, and it was tearing him apart, but he was also hurting himself. *'I feel lost,'* he said. *'I don't know who I am any more.'*

Mary then said, *'I'm angry and hurt, but I love him and want to help and support him as much as I can – also, he has no one but me.'*

After treatment:

After two sessions of Hypnoquit, Mary and Jim came back to see me for their final session. Jim was not viewing pornography at all. He told me he had completely lost the compulsion to go online and barely touched the computer these days. *'I have my life back,'* he smiled. Mary, too, was delighted, *'I've learnt through my Hypnoquit treatment to understand his addiction more. We're working through this together. I feel like I've got my husband back and we are spending more time together.'*

WHAT CAUSES A PORNOGRAPHY ADDICTION?

Pornography has no expectations and no emotions to deal with, and for some this is preferable to trying out the dating game: it's less trouble and effort, and you score every time! But of course this is not what we are meant to do. We are designed to have relationships with real intimacy, and all the complexities that go with this. But this can appear threatening to some people, so they search for 'intimacy' in less threatening places: pornography.

There is also a downward spiral, as with all addictions. After viewing pornography, your senses are dulled. You feel empty.

There is growing shame, a feeling of worthlessness, hopeless-ness and ultimately despair.

Pornography addiction can, in other words, be as devastat-ing to relationships and family life as any sexual addiction – indeed any other form of addiction.

Pornography addictions can also hurt other people emo-tionally, as the addicts are highly secretive. They tend to conceal their addiction – or they think they do – and this can destroy trust in relationships.

WHO BECOMES ADDICTED?

Studies show that men are more likely to view Internet pornog-raphy, whereas women are more likely to engage in erotic chat. Many people who become addicted to online sex have low self-esteem, or a distorted body image, untreated sexual dysfunction or a prior sexual addiction. But most people who become addicted to Internet sex have never had a problem with sex addiction at all. And many people view Internet pornography now and again, without any addiction to it whatsoever.

Help yourself by installing Internet filtering on your computer

Internet filtering software will block pornography websites on your computer. You therefore have to bypass your filter if you want to access these websites. The act of bypassing a filter can be a valuable 'stop sign' for you, allowing you to break the connection between impulse and action. It protects children too, if they use your computer.

HOW CAN HYPNOQUIT HELP YOU?

I am going to help you to overcome your chosen addiction to sex, pornography or Internet pornography. Using the daily meditations on the CD, you will quickly learn to separate your impulse to have compulsive sex, or to view pornography, from the action itself. This is because, with hypnosis, you will reach your subconscious mind – the part responsible for urges (see pages 208–10 for a full explanation of how hypnosis works to stop your urges).

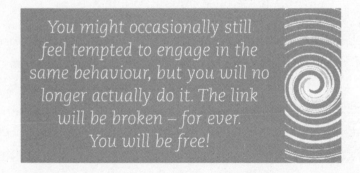

You might occasionally still feel tempted to engage in the same behaviour, but you will no longer actually do it. The link will be broken – for ever. You will be free!

At the same time, you will learn to identify your emotions and to feel more in touch with them. This will make you become more positive about life. As your self-esteem soars, you will lose the impulses that drive your addiction. You will find, without your addiction, that you have time and energy for life again: to do the things you love; to reconnect with the people you love; and to be yourself.

Sex will become for you a normal healthy part of any loving relationship, rather than an agonising, dehumanising addiction.

People tell me that losing their sex addiction through Hypnoquit is like getting their identity back: they feel like themselves again. They can hold their head up high, and love – and be loved – without secrets, lies or risks.

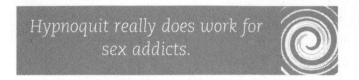

Hypnoquit really does work for sex addicts.

I have seen countless people – desperate, shamed and unhappy – who have come to me as a last resort and who have walked away liberated and strong. You can be one of them! It starts right here, right now.

Read Part 3, then use the action plan in Chapter 16 to get started.

8

IS THE INTERNET
CONTROLLING
YOUR LIFE?

The Internet has revolutionised the way we communicate, connect, learn, work and explore. Internet use has exploded in recent years, providing a constant and changing source of entertainment and information. It is an indispensable lifestyle tool. From Google and YouTube to MySpace, we now work, live, laugh and love online. You can also connect with hundreds of people on social networking sites such as Facebook or Twitter.

Television programmes such as *The X Factor* have increased the traffic on the networking sites, as people feel compelled to discuss their points of view and keep up to date with the contestants' private lives and antics.

Every day, new advances are being made in this amazing digital revolution. Three-quarters of UK homes have the Internet, and in 2010 alone we can look forward to 3-D TV and tablet computers. For many, the Internet is also an indispensable tool in the workplace.

WHEN IS IT TIME TO STOP?

In this high-pressure, 24/7-cyber society how much is too much Internet usage? Certainly, Internet addiction is the 'new kid on the block', when it comes to addictive behaviours. Some doctors are even arguing that it should be classed as a mental illness. Behavioural experts are increasingly united on one aspect: Internet addiction is fast becoming a serious public health issue.

In my clinics, in London, Europe and the US, I am seeing more and more clients who have become hooked on the Internet. Although it might appear to be a harmless medium to while away a couple of hours, overuse of the Internet resulting in addiction can be as devastating, as harmful and as overwhelming as an addiction to alcohol or cocaine.

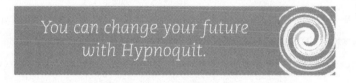

You can change your future with Hypnoquit.

HOW DOES INTERNET ADDICTION TAKE HOLD?

People who are addicted to the Internet spend unbelievable amounts of time online, as I've already explained with regard to Internet-pornography addiction in Chapter 7. An estimated one in five Internet addicts are engaged in some form of online sexual activity, but countless others are hooked, not on cybersex, but on the Internet as a whole, and they can become obsessed, trapped and desperate.

Some clients tell me that they can't stop checking emails,

compulsively using their BlackBerry, visiting social networking websites such as Facebook or updating and monitoring their Twitter account. Some have become obsessed with online gaming. Others are hooked on auction sites such as eBay where the high comes when you win a bid.

The opportunities are endless: booking holidays, theatre and cinema tickets, shopping websites such as asos.com, my-wardrobe.com and net-a-porter.com, or using the Internet to plan parties and venues and order food – and that's just for starters.

For many people, these shopping websites are a godsend and they wondered how they managed before Internet shopping, but there are others who become addicted. And that, of course, is where Hypnoquit comes in.

Some people simply become hooked on the search for information: checking, cross-checking and amassing information from endless sources. They justify this by believing that the information is work related, and often it is; however, with an Internet addiction, there is no real distinction between research for work or for personal reasons.

Breaking the rules

Internet addiction comes with a huge risk. It's quite extraordinary when you bear in mind that every employee is made fully aware of company policy on its use. Internet overuse often results in instant dismissal, yet those who are addicted still take the risk. This shows how addictions can take over and rule your life – until the day you decide to quit.

Questionnaire:
Are you addicted to the Internet?

	Yes	No
Do you need to spend increasing amounts of time online to feel satisfied?	☐	☐
Do you feel preoccupied with the Internet? (Do you think about your online activity or anticipate your next online session?)	☐	☐
Have you ever tried to cut down?	☐	☐
Do you feel depressed or angry when trying to cut down?	☐	☐
Have you lost opportunities or relationships because of the Internet?	☐	☐
Have you ever lied simply to hide how much time you spend online?	☐	☐
Do you use the Internet to escape from your problems?	☐	☐
Do you invariably stay online longer than intended?	☐	☐
Do you feel secretive when asked what you do online?	☐	☐
Do you feel that life would be boring or empty without the Internet?	☐	☐

If you answered yes to five or more of the above questions, you have an Internet problem.

Friends without socialising

Many of my clients tell me that they have made online 'friends' who feel more real to them than their actual social circle and, importantly, these so-called friends are non-critical. Some have committed a kind of virtual adultery, becoming highly emotionally involved with someone they have never actually met in the flesh. They spend so much time online that their career is suffering: they are online when they are supposed to be working. Their addiction is ruining their relationships, work life and mental well-being. And then one day, for a variety of reasons, they desperately want to stop, but can't.

Whatever the particular focus, these people have one thing in common: their Internet compulsion is taking over their lives. They have lost control.

> By reading this book you are one step towards regaining control of the life you were losing to the Internet.

★ **Case Study:** Harriet, a 31-year-old singer–songwriter, came to see me about her Internet addiction.

Before treatment:

'I was becoming increasingly despondent, waiting for my agent to secure work for me, and my song writing had dried up. I had writer's block, so I decided to surf the Net looking for inspiration. I even thought about changing my agent. I literally came across eBay by pure chance, as it was a pop-up *advert on one of the sites I was viewing. Of course, I had heard of eBay from my friends, but I'd never used it myself. I used to be too busy, but now my writer's block gave me more time to become mischievous.*

'I started buying things I didn't need. Most were cheap, so I thought I could give them away as presents if I didn't like them. I quickly became hooked on the bidding. I'd excitedly tell my friends that I seemed to win virtually every bid. I was proud of my achievements; it was as though I had got a new job and had excelled at it.

'It was quite interesting because in the past my friends used to tease me, saying, "Get into the modern world, Harriet, everyone's using eBay – we all do." But now they were more than concerned about how much time I was spending surfing the Net. I began to lie about how much time and money I spent online, and I became secretive about my bids. Then the penny dropped: I had a secret life. I was distancing myself increasingly from all my friends and spending too much time on my own with my computer as my friend. How ridiculous is that?'

After treatment:
I worked with Harriet to rediscover her self-confidence, self-esteem and self-worth. She was so keen to overcome this addiction and get her life back, because she felt it had been stolen from her by an inanimate object: her computer.

Harriet's story is by no means rare. It demonstrates how an innocuous curiosity can grab some people and change their life around. Hypnosis does the same: it changes your life around – but for the better.

> *As you follow Hypnoquit you will gain confidence and self-assurance to live without your addiction.*

WHO BECOMES ADDICTED?

Studies show that people who have other psychological issues, such as depression, anxiety disorders or obsessive-compulsive disorders are more likely to become addicted to the Internet. But actually, in my experience – and I see more and more Internet addicts in my clinic as the years go by – anyone can become hooked on the Web.

★ **Case Study:** Clinton, 59, is a CEO in a major financial institution. His addiction to the Internet started as the banking world crashed and he felt in danger of losing his job.

Before treatment:

Clinton knew that cuts were being made. Indeed, he was often the instigator. He used to be a statistician, and he was fully aware that it made sense to exchange a high salary – paid to just one man who was nearing retirement age – for a few senior managers. And any one of those senior managers, for all he knew, could have already been groomed to take over from him.

So, Clinton began surfing the Internet for other jobs, training courses and investments, but his behaviour became obsessive. He was absolutely astonished at his own weakness. He recalled reprimanding his 13-year-old son for spending too many hours playing games on his computer, and yet he, himself, was spending hours each day online and always at work.

His Internet addiction soon became out of control and he felt angry with himself, so he took steps to ensure he ended his addiction before he became one of his own statistics.

After treatment:

The Hypnoquit programme helped Clinton to overcome his addiction. He still goes online sometimes for work-related research, but he can control his behaviour now. He no longer feels the obsession to log on.

Common Internet addiction behaviours

There are some common threads when it comes to Internet addiction:

- **Using the Internet excessively,** losing sense of time, forgetting to eat and drink, and missing appointments when online. Addicts may lose sleep and neglect themselves physically because of the time and energy spent online.
- **Getting withdrawal symptoms.** Addicts feel angry, tense or depressed when they can't get online.
- **Being obsessed with the technology** – computers and software. Addicts want more and better equipment. Their computer feels like their best friend, their life.

HOW OTHERS SUFFER

I have seen the wider effects of an Internet addiction again and again, when my clients describe the stress it has placed on their loved ones. An Internet addiction is almost always damaging to family, work relationships and friendships.

You may argue with your partner about how much time you spend online. You try to conceal it. You may develop seemingly deep ties to other people in cyberspace, via chatrooms, 'second life' websites or social networking sites. You may lie about this too, or conceal it. You may get sucked into emotional situations you would have avoided in the real world. The website, Friends Reunited, for example, causes many relationship break-ups when old flames hook up and fall in love with the dream that was years ago. The problem is, of course, that this unsettles the existing relationship – and for what? Although some rekindled relationships do work out, most do not. In the meantime, hours and hours are spent furtively checking the website, 'talking' to the old flame, and reminiscing. It all feels more real, exciting and compelling than your real life. This gives you a high.

> *Recognising you have a problem is part of the battle towards beating it.*

PROBLEMS IN THE WORKPLACE

At work, you try to hide the fact that you are violating company policy by surfing the Internet, or using banned social networking sites (made possible because your 'friend' in IT has given you the passwords). You break the rules. You lie. You try to cover your tracks, but all that happens is you become more and more isolated, depressed and ashamed. You lie some more. The time you spend online and the secrecy surrounding this escalate. You're hooked.

Growing old too soon!

A recent report suggests that young people with excessive Internet use are becoming as isolated and lonely, and experience the same social problems, as the elderly, because they spend so much time on their own with their computer and away from family and friends.

★ **Case Study:** Tom, 34, a company secretary, who is married with two boys, was hiding a secret. He was bisexual, and he would surf the Internet for hours and hours at work, finding gay websites and chatrooms.

Before treatment:

Tom always arrived at the office early in order to log on, as he wouldn't risk this at home. Until one day, he arrived at work to discover a sticky note on his screen with one word on it: 'Homo'. He had his suspicions about who would want to show their disgust in this way, but the homophobe hadn't got the courage to disclose their identity; however, this was enough to send Tom into a spin.

He was mortified and felt physically sick. His brain went into overdrive and he felt panic-stricken. What about the shame on his family? And what if the local village

community, which he was heavily involved in, found out?
All this was so much of a shock to him that he resigned.

After treatment:
Tom sought my help, and was ultimately grateful to the
anonymous author of the note. It was his wake-up call.
Tom was always anxious at work, constantly worried that
someone would discover him using the chatrooms. Now,
with his addiction and his secret life behind him, he
feels calm and has found a new job.

 HYPNOQUIT tips
Find activities to replace the addiction:
- **Rebuild your life outside** this obsession with the Internet. It is
  ruining your life, causing you pain and also causing pain and
  anguish to those you love. To do this, it is important to find
  things that motivate you and excite you, and that get you
  outside – keeping you busy, interested and socially stimulated.
- **Find non-computer related activities** such as sports and
  hobbies. You'll reap the benefits when you increase your social
  circle, as well as becoming fitter and healthier through exercise.
- **Find sources of friendship** and activity in the 'real world'
  by looking at what interests you. Some of my clients join a
  hobby club, do some voluntary work, learn Salsa dancing,
  begin a creative writing or art class, or take up a regular sport.

TAKE INTERNET ADDICTION SERIOUSLY

It is important to take all computer addiction seriously, and not
to trivialise it. I've seen many people whose lives are almost

ruined by their Internet addiction. It really is a health hazard, both psychologically and socially, as it often involves an isolated, sedentary lifestyle.

Internet addicts also suffer many health-related problems. They forget how being outdoors is enjoyable, and how interacting with others can be fun and fulfilling.

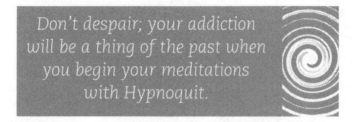

Don't despair; your addiction will be a thing of the past when you begin your meditations with Hypnoquit.

HOW CAN HYPNOQUIT HELP YOU?

Hypnoquit will enable you to quickly and effectively 'delete' the association in your mind between your emotions and needs and using the Internet. Using the daily meditations on the CD, you will quickly learn to ignore your impulse to use the computer unnecessarily.

Although you may still feel tempted to use the Internet when you don't need to, you will no longer do so because I will have broken the link in your subconscious mind. In its place you will enjoy the time you have now gained to pursue those interests that will make you happy and fulfilled in life.

Now is the time to learn again. Discover how Hypnoquit can help you to overcome the addiction so that you can live your life in the real world once more and have fun.

Read Part 3, then use the action plan in Chapter 16 to get started.

9

IS YOUR LIFE A HAZE OF CIGARETTE SMOKE?

You are undoubtedly aware of the facts, the statistics and the horror stories connected to smoking that have been passed on by the medical profession and the media, who regularly report the dangers of cigarettes. You might also have a friend or relative who is suffering, or who has died, from a smoking-related disease, and you now realise for yourself how dangerous smoking is. I am going to reinforce those messages, and I make no apologies for doing so; however, this time is different. You're reading this chapter because you want as much ammunition as possible to help you now that you have decided to quit. So, the facts and figures I'll be including here will ensure that you don't change your mind. This chapter contains more facts and figures than other chapters, but they are entirely necessary, as you will discover.

THE LOWDOWN ON CIGARETTE SMOKING

Tobacco use is the leading cause of preventable illness and premature death, and the World Health Organization (WHO) estimates that unless countries take drastic action, tobacco could kill about 8 million people every year by 2030, mostly in developing countries.

Smoking kills over 120,000 people prematurely in the UK every year. According to the WHO, smoking kills 5 million people around the world every year – that's more than 13 people every hour. Smokers will usually die 10 to 12 years younger than non-smokers. That makes for scary reading, don't you think?

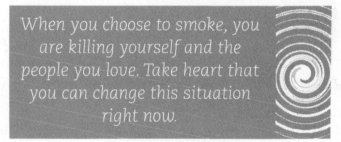

When you choose to smoke, you are killing yourself and the people you love. Take heart that you can change this situation right now.

FACT

Smoking tobacco products is the MAJOR cause of lung cancer, and it kills you and others.

THE SMOKING BAN

It is now against the law in the UK, Australia, New Zealand and in many states of the US and much of Europe, to smoke inside public places – cafés, clubs, pubs, shopping centres, bars, cabs and restaurants. Offices can no longer allocate an indoor smoking area. Even public transport and work vehicles used by more than one person are now smoke-free.

A significant number of young people are surprised to learn that smoking used to be allowed in commercial aeroplanes, cinemas, buses, trains (underground and overground), restaurants, offices, shops and virtually every public place. This is still acceptable and allowed in some countries! However, although the smoking ban has certainly spurred many people to give up smoking, there are always new young smokers taking up the habit every day. Smoking is not only a health hazard but it's also a major cause of fires in the home and is responsible for a significant amount of litter on our streets, especially since the smoking bans were introduced.

You may be one of the freezing, huddled individuals smoking outside your office, or popping out of the pub or restaurant every so often, missing out on conversation, warmth and conviviality to feed your addiction.

Surely it's time to quit?

Global statistics
- **Smoking and cancers** – The International Agency for Research on Cancer (IARC) states that tobacco smoking can cause cancers of all major organs; for example, the pancreas, stomach, liver, bladder, kidneys, cervix, bowel, ovaries and all upper respiratory cancers.
- **UK statistics** (from *Medical News Today*, March 2010) – according to the National Health Service (NHS) one-quarter of the adult population in the UK smokes (that's 20 million people). Smoking is the biggest cause of death in the UK; more than 120,000 smokers die every year. That is more deaths than the combined total of deaths from HIV,

illegal drug use, alcohol use, road traffic accidents, suicide and murders.

- **US statistics** (from *Medical News Today* March 2010) – according to the American Heart Association, 23.1 per cent of men smoke (24.8 million) and 18.3 per cent of women (21.1 million). According to the Center for Diseases Control and Prevention (CDC) an estimated 443,000 deaths occur every year in the USA from cigarette smoking, almost one in five deaths. As in the UK, that is more deaths than the combined total of deaths from HIV, illegal drug use, alcohol use, road traffic accidents, suicide and murders.

- **Australian statistics** (from Australian Council January 2010) – figures show that 18,000 Australians die prematurely because of smoking – that's 50 a day. Thirty per cent of men smoke and 27 per cent of women are regular smokers. Australia has approximately 5.3 million smokers. Out of 1,000 young Australian males who smoke, one will be murdered, 15 will be killed on the road and 250 will be killed prematurely by their tobacco smoking.

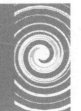

I have helped thousands of people to quit smoking over the past 23 years and they tell me it's like a miracle.

THE IMMEDIATE BENEFITS WHEN
YOU STOP SMOKING

The many health benefits from quitting smoking are evident from the moment you stop. You will begin to feel healthier, with more energy, and your skin tone will be glowing. What's more, your self-confidence will increase enormously. Don't just take my word for it, though; look at the following government statistics which apply when you stop smoking:

- **After 12 hours** many toxins such as carbon monoxide leave the body and you are able to breathe more easily. Energy levels increase and there is less strain on your heart.
- **After 2 weeks** your lungs begin to work better and the risk of heart attack decreases. Your circulation improves and you feel fitter.
- **After 3 months** the lungs have regained some of the capacity to clean themselves (providing there is no irreparable lung damage) and blood flow to the limbs will be improved.

Give up, don't cut down

Smoking raises your blood pressure and pulse rate for 20 minutes after each cigarette. Don't think, however, that if you smoke only a few a day your blood pressure and pulse will be OK and not badly affected; only by giving up and allowing your body to retain that normal level can you avoid serious illness.

DANGEROUS CHEMICALS

Tobacco smoke contains nicotine, which some experts suggest is as addictive as cocaine. But nicotine isn't the only dangerous substance; each cigarette contains more than 4,000 chemicals! Most are toxic and more than 60 are carcinogenic (meaning that they cause cancer). Here are some of the chemicals created when you smoke a cigarette; they make alarming reading:

- **Nicotine** – a poisonous alkaloid derived from tobacco, nicotine has highly addictive properties. It gets into the bloodstream and causes lung cancer and it stimulates the brain giving the 'rush' that keeps you hooked.
- **Hydrogen cyanide** is one of the many toxic by-products present in cigarette smoke. It is used to kill rats, and in the Second World War it was used as a weapon of mass destruction.
- **Carbon monoxide** easily combines with haemoglobin in the blood, causing breathing difficulties and putting a strain on your heart.
- **Tar** – every puff of tobacco smoke you take deposits tar into your lungs and causes lung disease. The tar in cigarettes contains carcinogens, which encourage the development of cancer in the body.
- **Formaldehyde,** used in glues and fungicides and to preserve dead bodies, is also present.
- **Benzene,** which is a chemical used mainly in the petroleum manufacturing process, is a known cause of acute myeloid leukaemia and kidney cancer.

Let's not forget the 260 dangerous ingredients in the paper, filter tip, ink for the monogram, whitener for the paper and the glue to hold it all together. Then, there is lighting the cigarette, which changes the chemicals, as it's burned at high temperatures; this carries its own health risks.

Although these dangerous chemicals are present in small quantities in each cigarette, you are taking them into your body several times a day.

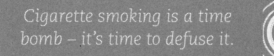

Cigarette smoking is a time bomb – it's time to defuse it.

CAN NICOTINE REPLACEMENT HELP YOU?

As you have seen, nicotine is a dangerous substance, but nicotine replacement products, which were intended to get you over the withdrawal problems of quitting smoking, are dangerous too. They were initially intended for short-term use, but often they are used for years. In fact, I have treated many people who have become addicted to them. And remember that nicotine is still getting into the bloodstream if you use replacements. There is a school of thought that believes nicotine does harm no matter how it is taken. Nicotine in the bloodstream remains the cause of lung cancer, and it can also have contraindications if you are pregnant.

Some scientists feel that certain nicotine replacement products do little harm when used in the short term – although others disagree, and the research continues – but don't become complacent about them. In my view it is far better to quit smoking without them, which is why hypnosis is preferable.

SECOND-HAND SMOKE

Passive smoking has always been one of my bugbears. Most smokers find it difficult to understand how their smoking habit can have a negative effect on those around them and that it can kill – it just takes a little longer to do so. Some smoking adults impose their habit on their own children, in their cars and in their homes. Although many parents recognise the dangers, far too many continue to expose their children to second-hand smoke (also known as environmental tobacco smoke, or ETS).

You may be unaware that second-hand smoke kills around 600,000 people around the world every year. ETS also contains the 4,000 toxic chemicals mentioned above, which can damage almost every organ in the human body. When exposed to your smoke, a non-smoker's risk of lung cancer goes up by 24 per cent. Their risk of heart disease rises by 25 per cent.

Smoking is an irritation to the lungs, as is ETS. It is undoubtedly linked to complications in asthma sufferers, causing more frequent asthma attacks. So, if you or your children or elderly relatives are asthma sufferers (a chronic disease) then you are giving them, and yourself, a precious gift by quitting.

On a personal note, I know how dangerous the effects of ETS can be, as I have developed respiratory illnesses, including asthma, purely from ETS. Even though I was acutely aware of the dangers and went to great lengths to avoid ETS, it still got me.

FACTS ────────────────────────────────

- Second-hand smoke can, and does, cause lung cancer, heart attacks, stroke and many other serious conditions.
- Children exposed to ETS can develop asthma – a chronic disease.

- Smoke travels around the house, so designating one room for smoking makes no real difference at all; smoke will eventually permeate the rest of the house. It's just like pouring chlorine into a pool at the deep end and expecting this to stay put and not circulate to the shallow end.
- Even low levels of ETS can cause health problems in non-smokers.

Wouldn't it be good to find a way to quickly and easily quit now, and for ever? The good news is, you have.

SMOKING IN THE CAR

There are other dangers too. I can never understand how a smoker can legally smoke while driving with one hand on the wheel and the other hand holding a cigarette. How do they change gear in a manual car? What happens if the lighted cigarette end drops into their lap? Strangely, although you can be fined for eating at the wheel in the UK it is not an offence to smoke. (However, there are currently rumblings about banning smoking while driving.)

All governments need to address these issues and turn those 'rumblings' into action before another family is killed on the roads through smoking. It has taken long enough to ban the use of mobile phones while driving. If smokers cannot see for themselves, which some clearly cannot, that smoking is dangerous while driving, then governments need to take action to protect everyone.

Take a moment to think about children placed in the smoky environment of a car. They have no choice or say in the matter; they're told to jump in the back and fasten their seat belts, but it's up to their parents to protect them, not just from road accidents but from health hazards too. This really is a very good reason in itself, to quit.

MORE GOOD REASONS TO QUIT

In case you're not quite convinced . . .

- There is enough nicotine in four to five cigarettes to kill the average adult if ingested whole; however, most smokers take in only one to two milligrams of nicotine from each cigarette because the remainder is burned off. (A manufactured cigarette contains approximately eight or nine milligrams of nicotine.)
- Passive smoking exposes you to more than 60 cancer-causing chemicals. Alarmingly, 11 of these are known to be Group 1 carcinogens (known to cause or aggravate cancer).
- Cigarette smoke contains low levels of radioactive lead and polonium (a lethal radioactive element that occurs naturally in very low concentrations in the earth's crust but is lethal in larger quantities – as the well-publicised death of Russian dissident Alexander Litvinenko demonstrates). You only have to check out the Litvinenko case on the Internet to discover how potent polonium is. The investigation into the contamination caused real panic. This may help you to understand how dangerous one of the chemicals in tobacco really is. And that's just one of many, as we have seen. According to a scientific report, some of the world's biggest

tobacco companies refuse to publish their research findings concerning the lethal radioactive substance polonium, because they fear litigation. Getting tobacco companies to face up to the damage they are doing is said to be 'like waking a sleeping giant'.

- Worldwide, one in four teenagers smoke cigarettes. This means that 80,000–100,000 kids start smoking every day worldwide.
- Despite all the publicity about its dangers, smoking will kill one billion people this century, unless serious anti-smoking efforts are made on a global level.
- Smoking is also responsible for erectile dysfunction (male impotence) in some cases. What man would want it known that he is unable to perform just because he smokes?

THE PHYSICAL EFFECTS OF SMOKING

Smoking causes many distressing illnesses:

- **Emphysema** is a type of chronic obstructive pulmonary disease (COPD) involving damage to the air sacs (alveoli) in the lungs. When this happens your body is unable to get the oxygen it needs, so you will struggle to breathe. Daily quality of life is arduous. The lung tissue loses its elasticity, the walls of the air sacs tear and stale air becomes trapped, eventually causing death from a lack of oxygen. This condition, along with lung cancer, is the most feared by the majority of smokers. There is no cure for emphysema, although in mild cases surgery can help.
- **Lung cancer** is the second most common cancer diagnosed in the UK. (Breast cancer is the most common cancer in women

and prostate cancer is the most common cancer in men. Smoking is one of the causes.) Every year around 40,000 people are diagnosed with lung cancer – that's 109 every day! It is the most common cancer in the world with 1.3 million people diagnosed in 2002. According to GLOBOCAN (Cancer Incidence and Mortality Worldwide) an estimated 12.7 million new cancer cases and 7.6 million deaths occurred in 2008. The most commonly diagnosed cancers worldwide are of the lungs.

- **Tobacco smoke** causes almost 90 per cent of all lung cancer deaths. One in ten heavy smokers will get lung cancer and in most cases it is fatal. Lung cancer is difficult to detect, and it's therefore likely to have spread to the liver, brain and bones by the time you seek medical help. Often the symptoms that have caused you to go to the doctor are from the secondaries (the sites the cancer has spread to). For this reason, lung cancer is known as the silent killer because it is often not discovered until it's too late.

FACT

Overall, less than 10 per cent of people with lung cancer survive for more than five years after diagnosis.

- **Heart disease** (called arteriosclerosis), is responsible for most heart attacks. Plaque, deposits of cholesterol, which collect in the coronary arteries narrow the blood vessels until eventually the oxygen supply to the heart is stopped. Smoking accelerates this process.
- **Gastric ulcer** – smoking undoubtedly increases the production of gastric juices, raising the acidity level and eroding the

stomach lining. Painful ulcers result from these eroded areas and increase the risk of haemorrhage and perforation of the stomach lining.

- **Foetal risk** – carbon monoxide in cigarette smoke reduces the oxygen level in the foetus (the unborn child's) blood. Nicotine restricts the blood flow from the mother to the foetus, resulting in low birth weight. Smoking also increases the risk of premature birth and infant death.

- **Bladder cancer** – chemicals from tobacco are absorbed into the bloodstream and leave the body through the urine. These cancer-causing chemicals are always in contact with the bladder, as it's a holding tank for liquid waste, increasing the risk of bladder cancer.

- **Chronic bronchitis** is an inflammation of the airways. When cigarette smoke is inhaled into the lungs it irritates the airways so that they produce mucus. This mucus blocks the airways making it difficult for a person to get air into their lungs, so breathing is difficult. Chronic bronchitis increases the risk of lung infections, so it is essential to seek medical help to clear this up urgently. Cigarette smoking is the most common cause of chronic bronchitis.

- **Mouth and throat cancer** – cancer-causing chemicals from tobacco products increase the risk of cancer of the lips, the throat, the tongue, cheeks and larynx (voice box). The removal of these cancers can be disfiguring and can result in the loss of the larynx. There can also be loss of the tongue, which means that you are unable to speak and cannot taste or eat food, because you have to feed yourself through a tube directly into your stomach.

- **Stroke** – as smoking is a major cause of arteriosclerosis, or hardening of the arteries, it is a chief cause of stroke. Strokes occur when one of the arteries of the brain becomes blocked, or ruptures and forms a blood clot or bleeds into the brain. Once brain tissue is destroyed it cannot be repaired.

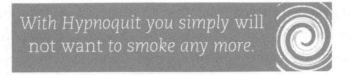

With Hypnoquit you simply will not want to smoke any more.

HOW THE ADDICTION WORKS ON THE BODY AND MIND

Cigarettes contain nicotine, a highly addictive substance found naturally in tobacco plants, which alters your brain chemicals. It is often said to be one of the most difficult addictions to overcome and, according to the experts, there is no way that tobacco would be legalised in most countries if it were introduced today.

When you inhale, the nicotine rushes to your brain where it affects two brain chemicals in particular: dopamine and noradrenaline. These brain chemicals alter your mood and attention levels, giving you that pleasurable, relaxed 'rush'.

This takes 16 seconds to achieve, so when you eagerly light up after a long-haul flight, for example, and feel better immediately, as you take in the first deep puff, it is not the nicotine that gives you the initial rush, it's the deep breath. So, after you quit, if you momentarily think you want a smoke (perhaps after a meal or when you have had a glass of wine), you are merely experiencing an association with smoking. Instead, take a deep breath and this will remove that supposed desire.

It's this feeling that you become addicted to. The more you

smoke, the more your brain becomes used to these chemical changes. You have to smoke more, to get the same feelings. You begin to crave cigarettes, more and more.

When you quit smoking, your brain chemicals are altered again, and with most methods you tend to feel anxious or depressed or quick to fly off the handle. You feel that only a cigarette will solve all this, so you crave it even more; however, with Hypnoquit, there are none of these usual side effects. You will feel calm, relaxed and very proud, because it is your involvement, determination and commitment, along with hypnosis, which will enable you to become a non-smoker easily.

★ **Case Study:** Gerry, 33, is an artist. He had smoked tobacco (about 20 a day) and cannabis since his teens.

Before treatment:

Gerry's girlfriend was giving him grief to stop. She is anti-smoking and, more importantly, she has severe asthma. Gerry felt that although he wanted to stop, he didn't like being forced into it by someone else. He told me,

'My girlfriend is oblivious to my feelings. She doesn't take into account how difficult it is to quit smoking, especially as I enjoy a joint every evening.'

Gerry did admit, however, that the cannabis had affected his memory. He became docile, got the munchies and ate unhealthily. He wanted to get back into shape and feel more alert. He was also keen to move in with his girlfriend, but she had given him an ultimatum: quit or stay in their respective apartments.

Once he had got past the issue of his girlfriend's pressure, Gerry did admit to me that he was becoming rather bored of smoking and the hold it had over him.

He said he'd like to stop, but he didn't think he could, as he had tried many different methods before. He had always promised himself that he would quit smoking before he reached 30. (Interestingly, a great percentage of my clients want to quit before their thirtieth birthday.) Gerry was three years late, but that's OK, you can't always predict when you will quit! But you will know when the desire to quit is there, and there will be no mistaking it.

After treatment:

Hypnoquit, coupled with the desire to stop smoking, was strong enough for Gerry to quit easily. After just one session with me he no longer craved either cigarettes or cannabis. Four months on, he told me he felt more alert and much healthier; he was producing better work, being punctual, getting some exercise and eating more healthily – and, yes you've guessed it, he was about to move in with his girlfriend.

Cannabis

Many young people try smoking cannabis at school, university or just because it's cool to smoke a joint, and all your friends do it so you naturally want to 'fit in'. You may give it a year or two and then become bored with it and stop as easily as you started; however, for others it is not so easy.

The main psychoactive ingredient in cannabis is delta-9-tetrahydrocannabinol (THC) and there are around 400 other chemicals in a cannabis plant. When you smoke a joint, THC rapidly passes from the lungs into the bloodstream, which carries the chemical to the brain. THC acts upon specific sites in the brain, called cannabinoid receptors, leading to the high; however, cannabis smoking has detrimental effects on the heart, lungs and brain.

So, although getting stoned may seem like fun, it has its consequences, as do all recreational drugs. Cannabis increases the heart rate by 20–50 per cent shortly after smoking, and this carries its own risks, especially with a person who has heart issues. Numerous studies have shown the effects of cannabis being an irritant to the lungs and it also contains carcinogens. According to the studies, cannabis smoke contains 50–70 per cent more carcinogens than tobacco smoke and, because cannabis smokers tend to inhale more deeply then tobacco smokers and hold their breath longer to get a better high, they increase the lungs' exposure for longer, so there is the potential for more damage. Having said that, other case-controlled studies have not found conclusive evidence to link cancer with smoking cannabis.

Smoking 'dope' is often used to relax, to forget problems, to meditate, to converse and to enhance creativity, to name a few. With long-term use, however, the opposite often happens: social interaction and life in general deteriorate and users become prone to depression and paranoia. Often people decide to quit just because they have used cannabis for a long time and decide it's time to quit and that they are tired of hanging around with other dope smokers. You have your reasons too and you will quit, easily and effectively, because you want to.

THE BENEFITS OF QUITTING

When you have followed the daily Hypnoquit meditations on the accompanying CD you will:

- Reduce your risk of death or serious health problems, such as cancer, heart or lung disease.
- Cut your risk of developing serious circulatory problems.
- Cut your children's risk of developing asthma.
- Have improved fertility.
- Enjoy food more, as your taste buds will be cleaner.
- Become fitter and have more energy.
- Smell fresh and your skin, teeth and hair will be healthier.
- Breathe more easily.

Start the meditations and your life as a smoker is finished – for ever.

 HYPNOQUIT tips

- Before you begin, make sure that you really want to quit smoking for yourself, rather than being pressurised by someone else.
- Choose a quit date, one that you expect to be as stress-free as possible.
- Calculate how much smoking costs you annually.
- Think of what you can or will buy with the money you are going to save.
- See yourself as a non-smoker when you quit.

HOW HYPNOQUIT WILL HELP YOU

You may think that smoking is something you'll never be able to quit, or that you certainly won't be able to do so easily, and you've probably tried many times before. You no doubt feel that it has a deep physical and psychological hold on you that is almost impossible to shake. You probably tell yourself, 'I've been smoking for too many years to be able to quit now', or 'It's too late for me, I have probably done all the damage I am going to do, so what's the point of quitting now?' But there is every reason to quit, and no possible reason to continue.

Anyone can quit smoking easily, and permanently, with Hypnoquit. The sooner you quit, the better the chance of repairing your body. And, as you have seen, the moment you quit, your body will begin to repair itself. There is strong scientific evidence that if you quit by the time you are 30 years old, you will repair most of the damage. But the sooner you quit the better – don't wait until it's too late. And remember that whenever you quit you can be sure that everyone – not only you – will benefit from your increased health and the longer life you will be giving yourself.

Using my meditations on the accompanying CD, you will simply 'delete' the urge to smoke from your subconscious mind.

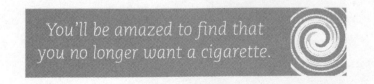

You'll be amazed to find that you no longer want a cigarette.

It's like a switch being turned off. From your very first Hypnoquit session you will feel happier and healthier, and free from cravings. Some people may need a few reinforcement sessions so, if you feel you need to, listen to the CD daily until you are comfortable to do without.

Read Part 3, then use the action plan in Chapter 16 to get started.

10

IS ALCOHOL TAKING OVER YOUR LIFE?

The majority of people enjoy an occasional drink of alcohol without it affecting their lives in any way. They may drink two or three times a week and will keep their consumption to well within the recommended weekly maximum levels; however, you may be surprised to learn that alcohol actually causes more harm in our society than illegal drugs such as heroin and cannabis. Every day there are countless alcohol-related accidents and illnesses that result in hospital admissions.

FACT

Alcohol abuse is costing the NHS in the UK £2.7 billion per annum and costs the US an estimated $220 billion per annum. The estimates for the cost of alcohol abuse in Australia range from $15 to $36 billion.

Alcohol abuse is a huge problem in the UK and worldwide. You may have seen the BBC programme *The Truth about Crime* filmed in Oxford, which showed how alcohol-fuelled violence puts a huge strain on the NHS, taking up the vast majority of police and A&E resources on Friday and Saturday nights.

Other countries have similar programmes. These programmes show the gruesome effects of alcohol addiction and misuse, and they are meant to shock. They show the major strain on the workload and resources of the NHS. There are scenes of mangled limbs, especially feet, as drunken teenagers collide with a vehicle while crossing a busy road, thinking they are invincible under the influence of alcohol. These images are horrific. Unbelievably, people repeat these same drunken patterns over and over again. Doctors and nurses show little sympathy.

I am not here to judge anyone, but simply to give you the facts and to help you to overcome your addiction. I will use every piece of ammunition in my armoury to do so, and if it means giving you gruesome details, then so be it.

The misconception that an alcoholic is someone who is always 'falling over drunk' on a daily basis couldn't be further from the truth. Many alcoholics are functioning alcoholics, and their colleagues and friends would be shocked to discover this.

THE TRUTH ABOUT ALCOHOL

You may have convinced yourself that with alcohol you

- Feel more confident.
- Have more fun.
- Are doing yourself no lasting harm.
- Are not alone, 'All my friends do it!'

Well, let's start with some facts about the effects of alcohol:

- One in ten adults and young people in the UK now drink too much alcohol – either from binge drinking, social drinking or alcohol dependence.
- Ten million people are abusing alcohol in the UK alone.
- Alcohol can damage your liver and brain: it causes cirrhosis of the liver and seriously affects your memory.
- Alcohol is linked to many cancers.
- Alcohol is linked to depression and suicide. It can cause homes, marriages and families to break up, and it destroys careers.
- New UK research indicates that between 3.4 and 3.5 million children now live with at least one binge-drinking parent.
- The World Health Organization (WHO) estimates that 76 million people worldwide suffer from alcohol-related disorders.

WHY MIGHT YOU BE ADDICTED TO ALCOHOL?

Drinking alcohol has profound physical effects on your body. Alcohol is a tranquilliser. Over time, it alters the balance of your brain chemicals, depleting some and increasing others. These changes cause a craving for alcohol and you gradually need to consume larger amounts to get the same sensations, the same highs. This becomes an addiction.

Have our genes got anything to do with it?

Some experts believe that alcoholism runs in families. Others disagree and believe that the environment and peer pressure is the main causes, which does make sense. Although either may be true, as an addict you don't need to know where your addiction came from – and you probably couldn't even care less – you simply want to stop it.

> *Hypnoquit is proven to be effective in helping people to free themselves from a dependency or damaging relationship with alcohol.*

Social, emotional and lifestyle factors

Alcohol addiction may have many complex causes. Many of the people I see are highly stressed. They are under pressure at work or at home and have increasingly taken refuge in alcohol. Many alcoholics have experienced past emotional pain or turmoil. Low self-esteem and depression are also common factors. Furthermore, if your partner is a heavy drinker, you may find yourself under pressure to drink more – or your drinking habit may be enabled by your partner's drinking.

Alcohol is one of the addictions that alters your personality: you usually talk non-stop nonsense or pick a fight, or flash your bits – or indeed all of these when you have reached the drunken state. Alcoholics, or even those who drink excessive amounts of alcohol – you don't have to be an alcoholic to suffer the negative effects of excess – can become belligerent, argumentative and sometimes violent. They take risks, such as driving when they have been drinking. The next day they are always sorry – until the next time, that is. Alcoholics can be promiscuous too, and I have heard of young girls waking up the next day with a stranger in their bed, with no idea how they got home or what has happened with this stranger.

Finally, there is the simple issue of availability. Today, alcohol is easy to buy and it's cheap: in some supermarkets a bottle of alcohol is cheaper than a bottle of water! And most adults and teenagers do drink alcohol, whether in moderation, frequently, very infrequently or addictively.

What type of person becomes addicted?

I have learned one key aspect from years of treating alcohol addictions: anyone who drinks alcohol, regardless of their background or age, can develop an addiction to it. Addiction usually happens gradually, a drink socially here and there. Many people who are addicted will be functioning alcoholics. As time goes on they begin to see the whole structure of their lives start to disintegrate.

★ **Case Study:** Sam, 54, and a marketing manager was a functioning alcoholic.

Before treatment:

Sam was in charge of marketing for a medium-sized software company. He travelled widely, worked very long hours, and socialised as part of his demanding job. He was often jet-lagged in hotels at unsociable hours, and gradually he'd find himself drinking alcohol to unwind.

Sam would often empty the hotel mini-bar. He'd drink on planes. He'd drink with clients. He'd drink alone with meals. Eventually, he was drinking two bottles of wine a day and sometimes a few glasses of champagne or spirits on top of this. But nobody knew he had a problem with alcohol – or if they noticed they certainly said nothing. Sam's performance at work was great. His team loved him. He was successful, he was gregarious and generous, especially when he had had a few drinks.

Inside, Sam was becoming increasingly desperate:
'I got so that I couldn't function without a drink and was preoccupied by it. I didn't feel human without a drink inside me. Then I'd be so tired – I'd excuse it as jet lag – but I'd be shaky and have this sick feeling. I was out of control and began to really worry when I found myself ordering a whisky on an 8.00 a.m. flight. I knew I was making myself ill and that I had to stop.'

Sam had a formal presentation to do and he suddenly felt nausea as he left his seat heading for the podium. He was nursing a hangover and his mind simply went blank. He felt exposed and vulnerable and decided then to seek help.

After treatment:
Sam quit completely within a few weeks using Hypnoquit, and his energy, work and social life changed beyond belief. He told me that he has never felt happier.

WHERE DOES SOCIAL DRINKING STOP AND ALCOHOLISM BEGIN?

It is incredibly easy to drink too much. Have you noticed how wine glasses in bars have got bigger? They are huge! We even pour ourselves huge glasses of wine at home at the end of a long day. We drink mega-strength beers in bars and pubs. What's more, rather than sipping a gin and tonic, or a vodka and orange juice or whisky with ice or water, we order shots of spirits and drink them back in one go. We invariably have no idea what a unit of alcohol is, or what constitutes a safe weekly limit. Social events and business meetings are structured around alcohol. I often hear of business meetings conducted around lunchtime, with excessive amounts of alcohol. Sometimes the participants go back to work even though they can hardly function, but they often don't bother going back at all and simply extend the meeting into a drinking session, carrying on well into the evening.

Today, teenagers see drinking to excess as fun and that every social occasion must include it. Whether this is from seeing their own parents drinking to excess or whether they are just copying what other teenagers do it is hard to say, but attitudes to drinking have certainly changed a great deal since the 1970s. The drinking culture among some young people is so prevalent that even before they are legally allowed to consume alcohol they are very likely to be drinking heavily, at least occasionally, when in the company of friends.

HOW MUCH ALCOHOL IS REASONABLE?

The easiest way to work out how much you are drinking is to count the units of alcohol:

1 unit is 10ml of pure alcohol: a standard pub measure of spirits, a half pint of normal-strength beer or lager, or a small glass of wine.

The recommended limit for women is 2 to 3 units per day, with a maximum of 14 units per week and one to two alcohol-free days per week.

The recommended limit for men is 3 to 4 units per day, with a maximum of 21 units per week and one to two alcohol-free days per week.

However, remember that some ale has an alcohol content of 3.5 per cent but stronger Continental lagers can have an alcohol content of 5 per cent or more, which equals 2.8 units of alcohol.

Don't forget the size of your glass too. Spirits used to be served in 25ml measures (1 unit of alcohol), but many bars now serve them in 35ml or 50ml measures, which is equal to 2 units. A large glass of wine is 250ml, which is one-third of a bottle and almost 3 units of alcohol in one glass, so your daily recommended limit would be just one glass with these measures. If you have three glasses of wine, you will have drunk a whole bottle without realising it. What is more, you would have had three times your daily limit.

Moderation vs bingeing

These 'safe limits' assume that your drinking is spread out through the week, not binged in one or two crazy nights out. There is some research that binge drinking a couple of times a week starts to kill off your brain cells. This is why UK government health advice says that a man should drink no more than 4 units in any one day and that a woman should drink no more than 3 units. (The Australian government advises drinking no more than two standard drinks on any day. In New Zealand the recommendation is six standard drinks for men and four standard drinks for women on any one day. A standard drink contains 10 grams of pure alcohol.) Of course, many people these days routinely drink more without realising it. If you drink a large glass of wine while cooking, you can easily consume 3 or 4 units. Another glass with your meal and you're at dangerous levels already. This leads to 'stealth alcoholism' as Rick, overleaf, found.

★ **Case Study** Rick, 40, works for a hedge fund and was addicted to alcohol.

Before treatment:

He is single and works long hours, socialising late into the night after work, as well as at weekends and when travelling.

'I started drinking when I went out after work. I'd have a few beers, and champagne to celebrate a deal, maybe some cocktails. I only actually got falling-down drunk a couple of times a month. But I'd drink a lot overall, steadily, throughout the week. I didn't get bad hangovers, and I was always on the ball at work. Sometimes I'd decide to not drink for a week or two, but before I knew it there'd be client meetings, or a deal and I'd be knocking back the cocktails. It was the lifestyle – everyone was doing it.

'It was when I couldn't stop drinking even on my "nights off" (in my flat, alone) that I knew it had gone too far. My friends and colleagues would be really surprised to know I had a problem with alcohol – I'm sure I appear perfectly normal to them. I've never messed up. I'm doing brilliantly at work and I function well. But I am addicted; this is bigger than me and I need help.'

After treatment:

Rick took just over three weeks to come off alcohol completely. He noticed his skin was healthier, and he was sharper and more alert. He joined a gym and began to take his fitness seriously. Rick always thought he was on the ball, but he was astonished to see his performance at work sky-rocket, and he told me that now he was looking forward to the rest of his life.

Questionnaire:
Are you an alcoholic?

Do any of these statements ring true for you?

	Yes	No
'I just don't feel right without a drink.'	☐	☐
'I can drink a lot without getting drunk.'	☐	☐
'I often drink on my own.'	☐	☐
'I need to drink more and more alcohol to get the same buzz.'	☐	☐
'I need a drink to start the day.'	☐	☐
'A few hours after my last drink I start to feel shaky, sweaty and tense.'	☐	☐
'I can't stop drinking even when I try.'	☐	☐
'I can't stop drinking even though I know drink is interfering with my career, my family and my relationships.'	☐	☐
'I get memory blanks where I can't remember what happened for hours or days.'	☐	☐
'I can't go for more than one day without a drink of alcohol.'	☐	☐

If any of these sound like your relationship with alcohol, they are the warning signs of alcohol abuse.

Hypnoquit is the answer to drinking that is spiralling out of control.

'BUT I AM NOT AN ALCOHOLIC'

Many people I see have a huge problem with alcohol. But they don't tick all the official boxes of alcoholism. Doctors call this 'alcohol abuse'. Basically, you drink excessively, you suffer health or social problems because of your drinking, but you aren't fully addicted, you still have some control.

If your drinking is negatively affecting your life, you do need to consider stopping, whether or not you think you're addicted. You can change your behaviour and liberate yourself. You can become healthier, happier and freer. And it's straightforward.

FACT

An alcoholic, or someone who is alcohol dependent, is defined as having all the symptoms listed above but they continue to drink despite all the problems alcohol causes them in their life, and they feel powerless to stop.

Important warning: alcohol

If you are **severely dependent** on alcohol – not a 'functioning alcoholic', but someone who drinks heavily every day – I strongly suggest that you seek medical guidance before embarking on the Hypnoquit programme, as you could be in danger of having a seizure or other serious side effects if you stop alcohol completely, when your body has been used to heavy drinking every day.

OVERCOME ALCOHOL ADDICTION FOR EVER

In addition to the daily meditations on the CD, which will stop your urge to drink, I suggest you begin an 'alcohol diary'. You may feel that you want to quit but are not quite ready yet. Keeping an alcohol diary will help you to make your decision sooner rather than later.

EXERCISE: keep an alcohol diary

All you need is a small notebook that you can carry with you at all times. Here's how it's done:

Use two pages for each day:

Page 1 note down the units of alcohol you drank and when.

Page 2 make a note of your general emotions throughout the day. Say, for example, if something annoys or upsets you so you feel the need for comfort and, in your mind, alcohol has always given you this, or if someone makes you feel happy so that you feel like celebrating.

You might be shocked by how much alcohol you do consume, even when you think you've hardly had anything. This can be a valuable wake-up call. By noting your emotions, too, it can help you to understand what prompts you to have a drink.

HYPNOQUIT tip
Use your diary *at the time*, not later

Always note down what you drank as soon as you have it, rather than trying to tot it up at the end of a day. This helps you to be more honest and also to remember how you were feeling at the time.

THE DANGERS OF ALCOHOL

Here is a sobering thought: friends are often amused by their drunken friend's antics, and when he or she passes out it causes even more amusement; however, alcohol irritates the lining of the stomach and can cause vomiting. The danger of choking to death on vomit and asphyxiation if you are not conscious (because of the intoxication) is a reality and is a risk you take every time you get drunk. There are many alcohol-related tragedies caused by asphyxiation, which could easily have been avoided.

> Hypnoquit can help you to release the grip alcohol has on your life.

There are so many myths surrounding sobering-up a drunk: strong black coffee, a cold bath or leaving the drunk to sleep it off. In fact, it is dangerous to assume that someone will be fine after they have slept. Many people fall into the trap of thinking that the drunken person will be fine in the morning. Although they may well be OK the next day, they might not wake up at all. Sadly, over the years, I have heard many stories from people who have regretted not seeking medical attention for a friend who had passed out through alcohol. They feel responsible for a tragedy which could have been prevented.

Critical signs of excessive alcohol

Vomiting is one of the first signs of drinking excessive alcohol and is a warning of alcohol poisoning, which can be very dangerous. Other signs that drinking has reached hazardous levels are:

- Seizures
- Hypothermia (abnormally low body temperature, shown by pale and bluish skin colour – this can be fatal)
- Mental confusion, coma or the inability to be roused
- Slow breathing (fewer than eight breaths per minute). The normal breathing rate is 18–20 breaths per minute

---

Alcohol poisoning is caused by drinking too much alcohol too quickly over a short period of time. On average, the human body can only process 1 unit of alcohol per hour (this varies slightly depending on many circumstances, including body weight). Many of the clients I have seen over the years will go out on a binge drinking session with the sole intention of getting drunk as quickly as possible. They are completely unaware of the dangers they place themselves in.

Alcohol is drunk by most adults, many of whom are responsible and respectable people. Most people believe it's a sociable thing to do and, because it is legal, it must therefore be OK. Of course, for most people it probably is, but for some it is not. You may be in either category.

RECOGNISING THE PROBLEM

So, by reading this you may well be beginning to face up to the problems you have with alcohol. This is your first step towards liberating yourself from the enormous physical danger and distress of alcoholism. Hypnoquit has helped thousands of people, just like you, to stop drinking and to regain a sense of calm and healthy balance. Using the daily meditations, you will find your cravings and your dependency simply melts away.

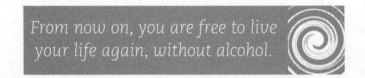

From now on, you are free to live your life again, without alcohol.

   Alcohol may be controlling you right now, but this can stop right here.

   Read Part 3, then use the action plan in Chapter 16 to get started.

11

HAS YOUR GRIP ON REALITY BEEN TAKEN OVER BY DRUGS?

Drug addiction is complicated and agonising, and it takes many forms. I see people who have become addicted to a range of substances, from cough medicine to cocaine, but what these clients all have in common is despair. They feel helpless, out of control and powerless, although initially the drug made them feel powerful and in control. They are now ruled by their addiction and they are risking everything for it. But they can't stop.

Drug addiction is a biological and pathological process that alters how the brain functions. Prolonged drug use changes the brain in fundamental ways, and invariably has long-lasting damaging effects on the brain and body. Even prescribed medicines can be addictive. This is why doctors are careful to monitor the period of medication and constantly review their patients.

THE DANGERS OF DRUG TAKING

Drug abuse is a frightening addiction because it is directly life threatening. Here are just some of the dangerous effects of drugs:

- Cocaine can cause heart failure.
- Heroin can cause respiratory failure.
- Cannabis can cause serious mental-health problems.
- Over-the-counter medicines can be fatal if misused.

When you read these facts, in black and white, you have to wonder why anyone would risk their life. But drug addiction isn't as simple as that, as anyone who has become addicted to prescribed medication or recreational drugs will tell you. Most people say their habit began tentatively. It gradually took hold, developing into a full-blown addiction.

ADDICTION TO MEDICATION

Drug addiction is insidious. It can start out with a simple course of medication to get rid of the symptoms associated with a genuine medical condition, and then develop from there.

Some medical conditions require long-term use of medication (for instance, inhalers for asthma or insulin injections for diabetes). These medications, if controlled, will save your life, not end it. Other medication, however, does not have to be taken in the long term: you treat the condition, then you stop taking the drug. An addiction can begin when someone continues to take this short-term treatment after its effects have been achieved. A long-term drug user can advance on to other drugs, such as sleeping aids or narcotic painkillers. This can lead to drug addiction.

Drug addiction causes huge heartache. Marriages and families break down because of it. My clients tell me how they have lost their friends, jobs, relationships, motivation and ambition. They become unreliable, irrational and know they are risking everything by continuing to misuse drugs – but they are powerless. The addiction calls the shots.

> You are no longer powerless;
> with Hypnoquit you can
> conquer your addiction.

★ **Case Study:** Anna, 34, works in the media and was addicted to cocaine.

Before treatment:

Anna came to see me, on the advice of a friend, because she knew she'd lost control of her cocaine use.

'I know I have to stop using cocaine, but I've been in denial, I just didn't want to face it. I know it's got out of hand. I just started using at parties. Everyone is doing it, after all. Well, everyone I know.

'I loved the buzz at first and the feeling of confidence I got from it. I began to party more and more and it was freely available, so I always took some. After I've had a couple of lines, I buy a few grams for me and my friends. I like to be the "powerful one" – as though I can afford to feed everyone else's appetite for cocaine, but in reality I cannot. It doesn't help that many of my clients also use "Charlie".

'I began to feel the effects were more and more short lived,

*so I had to take more to get the same buzz. Now I'm doing it
most days and seemingly can't function or face anyone without
it. I am in big trouble; socially, physically and financially and, of
course, I can't tell my family why. My friends are all worried
about me and they say they barely recognise me.*

*'I've lost a lot of weight, and I know I look terrible – I feel
really ill, out of shape and very down – and I'm starting to have
regular panic attacks. I know I have to stop before it's too late. I
am puzzled, though, as I didn't take more than my friends in
the beginning and yet I became addicted and they didn't.'*

After treatment:

Anna was very keen to get her life back. She said that she is
horrified to think of how far down she had sunk before
finding a method that helped her. Anna quit after just four
sessions and quickly got her life back to normal. She
remarked how impressed she was with the whole process.

HOW DOES DRUG ADDICTION AFFECT YOU?

Drugs are substances or chemicals that change the way our
bodies work. When you put them into your body, usually by
swallowing, injecting or inhaling them, they are carried through
the bloodstream to the brain where they alter your mood. They
either dull or intensify your senses, or they decrease physical
pain, make you happy, make you sad, or make you paranoid or
neurotic. Any one or more of these changes takes place. If the
experience was a pleasure, then you want more and a user
becomes an addict. If the experience was not pleasurable, but it
took away any anxieties, addiction is still a strong possibility.

Ultimately, drugs harm the brain and the body, and some drugs impair your ability to make good healthy choices and decisions in your life, causing innumerable problems.

When drugs take hold

- You lose interest in the things that you used to love; you lose motivation, drive and your *joie de vivre*.
- Your appetite changes (you either lose or gain weight).
- Your performance at work suffers.
- You feel moody, defensive, depressed and despairing.
- You become more secretive and dishonest, lying to friends, family and colleagues.
- You conceal your habit, and sometimes steal to fund it.
- You develop money problems.
- You lose your sex drive or become highly sexed/promiscuous.
- You become unreliable.

COMMON ADDICTIONS

Here are a few of the more common drugs that people become addicted to.

Cocaine

This highly addictive drug attacks the central nervous system and addiction often starts with people just trying it out. My clients (like Anna) generally tell me that they were offered cocaine with alcohol at a party (these twin addictions seem to go hand in hand). At first, they loved the buzz. It gave them a quick high, helped them to stay awake for an all-night drinking session and it made them feel more confident, more attractive and more sociable. It was fun and they had an intense feeling of power and energy.

For some people, such forays into the cocaine world are a rare indulgence. But for an alarming number of others, the buzz becomes a need, a way of life, an addiction. Cocaine calls the shots – not you – and even after one line, some people do develop physical and psychological cravings and find it difficult, if not impossible, to quit. They go on to spend a fortune on the drug, risking everything for it, and almost killing themselves in the process.

Cocaine is socially the drug of choice for many young successful partygoers.

FACTS

- Cocaine elevates the heart rate and blood pressure, and it can lead to death.
- Drug abuse can lead to prostitution, burglaries and street robbery to fund the addiction.
- The street value of all drugs has never been cheaper, as the supply outstrips the demand.
- Some users become attracted to making a living from dealing drugs and having a constant supply for themselves.
- In England and Wales, an estimated 2,000 people die every year because of illegal drug abuse.

Prescription drugs

This addiction often creeps up on you. A doctor prescribes you medication for a run-of-the-mill health problem – perhaps a painkiller for a back injury or sleeping pills for those sleepless nights. The medication brings with it not just a release from pain (or a good night's sleep), but a sense of well-being and relaxation. You feel better overall when you take it. As your medical condition improves, you keep taking the drug because it makes you feel so good. Soon, you need more and more of the medication in order to get the same feeling of well-being.

Before you know it, you are lying to your doctor, or buying the medication from the Internet. You're hooked. Sometimes people become hooked on prescription drugs that have not been prescribed for them.

There are countless risks associated with the prolonged use of prescription drugs and they include: damage to your digestive system, lungs, liver and kidneys and other internal organs. You may get side effects such as breathing difficulties, an accelerated heart rate or seizures. Remember that prescription medication can kill.

Drugs that are meant to save life can end it

The legendary Michael Jackson sadly died after abusing prescription drugs. He is by no means the only person to have died like this. Prescription drug abuse is endemic in our society. It causes huge pain and heartache, and many deaths.

Over-the-counter drugs

Myth An over-the-counter drug is safe or it would only be available on prescription.

Reality There is no such thing as risk-free medication.

The risks of abusing drugs that you can buy without a prescription are numerous and serious. Say, for example, that you are taking prescribed medication. You may accidentally overdose because some of the drugs you are buying over the counter may contain the same medication as the prescribed drugs you are already taking without you being aware of this.

This situation is horrendously common. The New York City medical examiner announced on 6 February 2008 that the young, talented Hollywood actor Heath Ledger died, tragically, from an accidental overdose of seemingly harmless medication, including commonly used over-the-counter sleep aids and pain relief.

Different countries have different regulations about over-the-counter drugs; for example, some drugs that are available only on prescription in the UK (such as certain sleeping aids and painkillers) can be bought off the shelves in US pharmacies in virtually any quantity you want.

I find that teenagers, particularly, tend to abuse over-the-counter drugs. One common form of medication regularly abused by teens is dextromethorphan (DXM), found in cough medicine and cold remedies. Alarmingly, many of the young people I see tell me that they were buying large quantities of DXM in powder form off the Internet and snorting it.

There are even websites that encourage children to share their DXM experiences. Such apparently 'harmless' medication is turning our children into drug addicts and should be stopped or regulated at the very least. Why are cough medicines and cold remedies not on prescription? We need to protect our children from themselves.

FACT

Large doses of DXM cause paranoia, vomiting, slurred speech, dizziness, seizures and death.

In short, there is no such thing as a safe drug.

★ **Case Study:** Georgia, 43, was addicted to anti-anxiety medication and sleeping pills.

Before treatment:

Georgia is a highly successful advertising executive, with three children, a happy marriage and, in her words, a 'beautiful home'. Her prescription-drug addiction spiralled after she began to experience panic attacks.

'The first time it happened I was going into an important meeting, and I just felt everything go black – like someone had drawn the curtains. I've always been able to cope, and I pride myself on having it all – doing everything brilliantly, giving everything 100 per cent: my children, my marriage, my job, my home, my appearance. It's very full-on keeping on top of it all, but I do. Or I did. I think it was like an overloaded computer; I just went into shutdown that day. Then I started shaking and couldn't breathe properly.

'I talked to my GP and she prescribed me some anti-anxiety

medication to help me through a particularly busy phase at work. Later, she prescribed some sleeping aids too. It escalated from there. The medications were effective and they got me through difficult phases. At first, I didn't take them all the time, by any means. But slowly I began to rely on them more and more until I was taking more than the recommended dose, and taking it every day – to wind down, to get myself through a stressful meeting or a difficult conversation, or just to get myself through life, generally.'

After treatment:

'With Hypnoquit, I didn't just kick the prescription drugs that were ruling my life, I also took a step back from it all. I realised the enormous pressure I'd put myself under to be perfect. I realised I didn't need to be perfect and that being "good enough" in some areas was OK. It was like taking a huge weight off myself. I know I'll never go back to those medications. It scares me how easy it was to get hooked, though. I thought they were "safe" – they came from the doctor, for goodness sake! What could be safer? But they almost ruined my life.'

Amphetamines

Prescription diet pills come under the category of amphetamines and I have treated thousands of people who have been happily taking these for years. (In fact, I would say that approximately half of all the clients I have treated over the years have tried diet pills.) As Sally told me,

'They kept my weight down and they were prescribed, so they must be safe. They gave me incredible amounts of energy. I couldn't sleep, and it was so funny because I just wanted to clean my home.'

Interestingly, many didn't seem to know that they were actually taking amphetamines. These stimulants accelerate the functions in the brain and body. They are sold in pill form and when sold as recreational drugs are known as speed.

Effects Amphetamines quickly produce a high and make the user feel energised, wired, powerful and alert.

Dangers They increase the heart rate and blood pressure, and breathing is difficult. Sleeplessness, headaches and shaking are also side effects. Prolonged use can invariably cause paranoia and, as they are addictive, if you stop taking them, anxiety follows and a craving for the drug develops.

There are still a few doctors who prescribe this illegal drug for slimming although it appears that they are now making their patients aware of the symptoms, but it doesn't stop patients who are so desperate to lose weight. And, of course, the user becomes addicted and wants more. In my experience it is not unusual for people to attempt anything to get slim, even following appalling diets that cause sticky blood, hair thinning, brittle bones and an early menopause. Often the users know the facts but still continue – so strong is their desire to lose their excess weight.

Questionnaire:
Are you addicted to drugs?

	Yes	No
Do you need more and more of the drug to get the same high?	☐	☐
Do you feel you rely on the drug, emotionally or physically?	☐	☐
Do you feel panicky at the thought of not having it?	☐	☐
Do you get withdrawal symptoms if you suddenly stop taking it?	☐	☐
Do you feel demotivated, or more negative and down, about life in general?	☐	☐
Do you feel that your performance at work or school is suffering?	☐	☐
Do you have relationship problems that are linked to the drugs?	☐	☐
Do you borrow or steal money to fund the drugs?	☐	☐
Do you lie about how much you use, or conceal your habits from loved ones?	☐	☐

If you have answered yes to more than three of these questions, you have a drug problem.

Hypnoquit is a proven method of breaking the hold that drugs have on your life.

HYPNOQUIT tips

Conquer your drug addiction

- **Avoid people who still use drugs.** This may seem obvious, but there is always someone in your old drug circle who would want you to fail in your quest to overcome your addiction. They don't want you to succeed where they have failed.
- **Never give up trying to quit.** Some people find that they can quit easier than others and some may relapse. If you relapse (this is highly unlikely, but not impossible) try again. Listen to the CD.
- **Listen to the CD** every day, until you feel you have conquered your addiction.
- **Enlist loved ones:** get friends and family to support you in your recovery and to offer reassurance when needed.
- **Get rid of the drugs.** Never save some for 'just in case'; this would be accepting defeat before you have even started.
- **Prepare for the difficulties** that may lie ahead. You may miss your old routine and addiction at times. You may not, but if you are prepared for this, there's no need to be afraid.
- **Stay active:** go for walks, take up a hobby, play sports – anything you love. Your addiction probably took up a big chunk of your time. It's important to fill that time with something you enjoy.

THE SIDE EFFECTS OF QUITTING

Drug dependence means that you need a drug to function normally. Abruptly stopping that drug generates side effects, some of which are more serious than others.

The extent of any side effects after quitting will depend on the drug itself and the length and severity of the addiction. Quitting cocaine, for example, can cause irritability, restlessness, depression and increased appetite (cocaine use suppresses appetite). On a positive note, you will have fewer nose bleeds and the liver won't have to work so hard to remove those toxins from the body.

Quitting cocaine

Apply the strict 'no use' rule, as it is easier than the indecisive cutting down 'Should I or shouldn't I get high one last time?' Over the years, my clients have told me how easily they quit. That's not to say that some of you may struggle for a few days and will need to listen to the CD more than your friends, for example, but don't measure your success against others. Quitting is the important part and not how you quit.

It is fair to say that of all the addictions I have treated, this is the one where a client invariably recommends Hypnoquit to a string of their friends who also want to quit. When one person quits, the gang does too, and especially when they discover how easy it was to do so.

Because alcohol can be a strong trigger for cocaine, give up alcohol for a few weeks too – in fact, the longer you can do this the better for your body to detox. Remember to quit any other drugs too, such as marijuana. Be in that mindset when you listen to the CD, and quit all recreational drugs. Quitting takes determination and effort, and you can do this with the support of family and friends (see Chapter 13) and with the help of Hypnoquit.

You may well experience what you believe to be 'cravings' for a few days after you quit, and you may see these strong urges as failure on your part or think that you will never be able to quit. If this happens, listen to your CD to reinforce the messages. Remember that you are simply experiencing a trigger, such as stress, boredom, loneliness or feeling sexually aroused, or you may be around the friends who use cocaine or who are talking about using. (In the earlier stages of using cocaine you felt highly sexual and this developed with further usage into not being able 'to perform', but you seem to remember the earlier stages and want this again.) The more aware you are of your triggers the better you are able to deal with them.

Remember that however unpleasant the side effects may be when you are enduring them, the rewards and getting your life back will more than make up for them.

Drug addiction can be complicated, deep-seated and very difficult to kick. But I have helped thousands of people, just like you, quit all types of drugs. You really can do this, no matter how much your addiction is currently ruling your life.

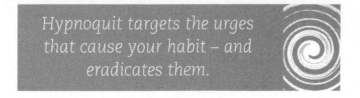

Hypnoquit targets the urges that cause your habit – and eradicates them.

If you practise the daily meditations, and if you really want to do this, then you can. It's not a miracle, although clients tell me it feels that way sometimes!

Read Part 3, then use the action plan in Chapter 16 to get started.

Important warning: drugs

If you are severely dependent on any drugs, whether
prescription (such as antidepressants and tranquillisers) or
recreational, I strongly urge you to seek medical guidance
and to use the Hypnoquit programme to simply support you.
You could be in danger of serious side effects if you stop
drugs abruptly and especially in an uncontrolled environment.
You may need residential treatment and counselling for
quitting heavy drug use, where you will be treated with
empathy and respect.

12

ARE YOUR RELATIONSHIPS AND YOUR HAPPINESS AFFECTED BY GAMBLING?

It probably started innocently. Perhaps a trip to a casino after a night out, a flutter on the horses, a fun way to pass the time online, but now you are unable to control your urge to gamble. You can't stop even though you are facing financial ruin and it's taking up valuable time. And you can't stop even though your family is begging you to.

Gambling is about risk taking. The anticipation and thrill you get when you make or win a bet gives you a buzz – one that's just as powerful as any high from drugs or alcohol, or any of the substances you'd normally associate with addiction. The more you gamble, however, the more addicted you become to this high. It helps you to forget your day-to-day life. It gives you an outlet, an escape, a distraction.

It also probably puts a huge strain on the rest of your life, whether that's family, marriage, relationships, finances, career or all of these. This, in turn, causes you to feel depressed and powerless. You probably dislike yourself at times for what you are doing. You then turn to gambling again, in order to escape the stress and self-loathing. It's a vicious circle, and you're stuck in it.

FACT ——————————————————————————————

The rates of attempted suicide among gambling addicts are at least double the national average.

You are not alone in your addiction, however. The addiction to gambling has become the fastest growing addiction in the UK. We now spend around £7.8 billion every year on gambling in the UK. The government estimates that around 350,000 people in the UK are addicted to gambling. Of these people, only about 5 per cent actually ask for help.

WHEN YOU REALISE YOUR GAMBLING IS A PROBLEM

In buying this book you may be one of the 5 per cent mentioned above, or you may have bought it for another reason and stumbled across this chapter. You might have read it out of curiosity only to discover that you or your partner is also addicted to gambling but that you have been kidding yourself it's just a hobby.

As with most addictions, you may have been in denial about this one. But realising that you have a problem is a large part of the battle. Now you can become one of the success stories by following Hypnoquit and leaving your gambling addiction behind you.

I have treated thousands of gamblers and helped them to quit for ever.

SOME PEOPLE JUST CAN'T GAMBLE RESPONSIBLY

'The House always wins', is a saying in Las Vegas, and most of us know this is true. Some people can gamble responsibly and enjoy it – a weekly lottery ticket, a game of bingo, the occasional flutter at the races or a little casino fun on holidays. Other people, such as Lisa below, however, simply do not fit into this category.

★ **Case Study:** Lisa, 33, came to see me about her gambling problems.

Before treatment:

As is often the case, Lisa's addiction started quite innocuously. She and her friends loved to go to the local pub and have a contest on the one-armed bandits to see who could win the jackpot first. It was rare that anyone actually won the jackpot, but that didn't stop them. Lisa would regularly put more than half of her wages into the machines. She'd think nothing of it. Her parents were generous and would top up her wages, although they didn't know why she ran out of money so often.

Fifteen years later, Lisa has advanced to Internet gambling and casinos, and she has upped her spending considerably.

'I can spend anything from £100 to £5,000 – all on credit cards – but I feel really powerful when I am in the casino. I

feel that I've come a long way in life, and can afford to spend as much as I want. I can't, of course – it's all on credit cards and loans. I get carried away with the thrill of the atmosphere, all that gambling and celebrating (to me, it always seems like gamblers are celebrating). I'll gamble all night, getting home at 5.00 a.m. when I have run out of money. I usually lose more in the casinos than at home alone on the Internet. I still lose track of reality when I'm Internet gambling, but I have no one else celebrating, so I'm not carried along with the whole excitement of being amongst other gamblers.

'One day I had a big loss, over £10,000. I felt trapped. I was in a mess and didn't dare tell anyone; because I'd lied to cover my tracks so much, no one had a clue how bad it was. I knew I'd let all my family and friends down. I seriously thought about killing myself, as it seemed like the only way out. I knew I couldn't borrow any more and I was running on empty in every sense.

'I had heard about Hypnoquit, and at first I thought Why would I need that? I thought I could control my own life, thank you very much. Obviously, I couldn't.'

After treatment:

'So I began a journey of life discovery. I decided that I wanted to know about me, about gambling, about why I had managed to become addicted. Why I had spent most of my parent's life savings, my ex-partner's "rainy day stash", why I'd ruined every relationship, lost good jobs and ended up with everyone avoiding me and seeing me as trouble.

'However, I understand now, because the programme has helped me to see clearly and to not apportion blame but to

just deal with it. I don't want to be complacent or even celebrate too soon, but I'm optimistic that I'm quitting gambling almost as easily as I became addicted. I am delighted. I find it interesting that I have come full circle. I've lost 15 years, but I am learning not to dwell on that. I am learning to live in the present and to put the past behind me, as I can't change it.

'Hypnoquit is teaching me that I mustn't waste energy on things I cannot change. I'm living in the present, but the future for me is exciting too, because I have never experienced adult life without an addiction. I've jumped from being a teenager to being in my thirties with no anecdotes about my life to be proud of and to share with others. But Hypnoquit isn't about looking back, or regrets, and I'm grateful for that – I'm happy and looking forward to the rest of my life.'

WHO BECOMES A GAMBLING ADDICT?

Statistically, men are more likely to become addicted to gambling than women, possibly because the gambling environment is more male dominated, but I do treat numerous women too, of all ages. The recent rise in Internet gambling is causing more and more women these days to become compulsive gamblers. There is also a link with alcoholism: around 50 per cent of gambling addicts are also addicted to alcohol.

INTERNET GAMBLING

Online casinos are a multimillion-dollar business. They don't just give existing gamblers a highly accessible outlet for their habit but they also pull in a new type of gambler: the person who might never have set foot in a casino or a betting shop, but who becomes hooked in the privacy of their own home.

When you gamble online it's easy to pretend that you haven't really lost much. It's also easy to exaggerate your possible winnings. It's just you and your screen. And in the anonymity of your home, you feel truly unaccountable.

You seem to overlook the fact that you have lost more than you have won. You simply remember and congratulate yourself on your winnings; that is, until more and more debt drops through your letterbox as you max out your credit cards. Then depression sets in. Yet you still believe you can win again to pay off those debts.

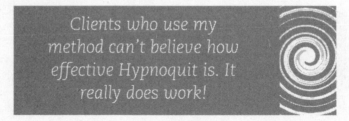

Clients who use my method can't believe how effective Hypnoquit is. It really does work!

You become secretive and can easily hide what you are doing. You can – and do – spend hours at your screen, losing thousands in the process. But you might do this when nobody is around, late at night perhaps, when nobody knows what you're up to.

When you finally see the light of day, you seek help. 'Thank God!' I hear your nearest and dearest shout. And this is where Hypnoquit comes in: you can stop this addiction right here, right now.

Clients tell me the Hypnoquit process is easy and amazingly quick, and they just lose the urge to bet.

Questionnaire:
Are you addicted to gambling?

	Yes	No
Do you spend more and more money to get the same thrill?	☐	☐
Do you lose work time because of gambling?	☐	☐
Do you gamble to pay off your debts?	☐	☐
Do you feel preoccupied with the next bet or gambling session?	☐	☐
Do you try to stop or cut down but can't?	☐	☐
Do you feel restless or irritable when you're trying to cut down?	☐	☐
Do you lose a bet, then go straight back to gambling again, trying to recoup that loss?	☐	☐
Do you see gambling as an escape or an outlet for stress or boredom?	☐	☐
Are you jeopardising your relationships or career by gambling?	☐	☐
Do you celebrate good news with a bet?	☐	☐
Do you struggle to finance your habit, or engage in illegal acts such as fraud or theft to finance it?	☐	☐

If the answer to more than three of these is 'yes', then you have a gambling problem. Hypnoquit can help you.

The different types of gambling

In our modern world, gambling is available virtually everywhere you look: on vacation or when you do your daily or weekly shopping. It can be found in subtle, and sometimes not so subtle, places.

- **Soft gambling** such as lotteries, scratch cards and bingo cards are available in virtually every supermarket, newsagent's and cruise ship, and in most holiday resorts.
- **Casinos** found in holiday resorts, towns and cities, and online.
- **Modern media gambling** available on the Internet, via interactive television and mobile phones.
- **Slot machines** found on cruise ships and in bars, pubs and arcades.
- **Dog tracks** found in some towns and cities.
- **Horse racing** held at racecourses around the country.

THE IMPACT ON FAMILY AND RELATIONSHIPS

Gambling can have a devastating effect on your family and on relationships with loved ones and friends. Usually, your immediate family will suffer most as they try to manage with less income while your gambling gets more and more destructive and you become more moody. People who love you will still find it difficult to live with you at times and find it hard to understand how you can seemingly destroy yourself and your loved ones as a result of your gambling.

★ **Case Study:** Brian, 28, is a father of two. He was just 14 when his gambling started.

Before treatment:

Brian's father took him to his favourite place – the dog track – which his father saw as a hobby. Dad said it was Brian's birthday present and gave him money to bet. He was proud to teach his son 'how it's done'. Unfortunately, Brian won a fair amount of money, known as 'beginner's luck'. It is amazing how many of my clients' gambling addictions began this way.

Over the years, Brian advanced to casinos, while becoming hooked on scratch cards, the lottery and fruit machines.

He had always been interested in computers but never any form of gambling online. He had a job, which paid well, so he had more disposable income and very few living expenses, as he was living with his parents. He lost all track of how much he was losing.

Over the years though, Brian's life changed dramatically, and for the better in some respects, but his addiction did not and it secretly spiralled out of control. He got married and had two children, but he was increasingly spending more time and money at the casino, just a short walk from his work.

One day he spent his entire month's wages in one afternoon at the casino. He was forced to get a loan from the bank, and acquired a number of credit cards.

'I promised myself that I would stop gambling when I got married, and then when each child was born, and then when my dad got sick but, of course, I didn't. I couldn't, and I knew I was kidding myself and needed help even then, but I just kept telling

myself that I would have one more month of gambling to recoup my losses. I told myself, "I only need one big win, then I'll quit."'

The big win never came for Brian. He was eventually declared bankrupt at 27. His wife walked out on him, taking the children with her. He struggled for a while to cope with his crippling and ongoing addiction. Then his flat was repossessed. He went back to his parents.

'I sat in my old bedroom with my good memories of a time when I would laugh with my friends, play computer games and exchange stories, and I didn't have a care in the world. I realised I had totally screwed up my life. This was rock bottom. I just howled for what seemed like hours.

'I believed that there was no way I could sort this out on my own, if at all. My parents were always a huge support, and mum had suggested hypnosis. She always has my best interests at heart and, after all, to me my mum is the "oracle" and I trusted her.'

After treatment:

Brian quickly overcame his addiction using Hypnoquit. He is still trying to deal with his personal issues, because his wife is naturally apprehensive, but they are talking and being parents, which is new to Brian. At our third and final session, he said: *'I feel as though I am just starting my adult life. I've somehow lost over ten years, but I don't live in the past, just the present and the future from now on.'*

Brian knows he has to take one step at a time. He knows his daily meditations are vital, and he also knows that he will never be complacent and think he can make just one bet. Brian has never felt stronger.

Remember

You might have a big win, but sooner or later you will lose it all again. Hypnoquit removes the temptation to keep repeating the pattern.

Note: some people can have that one big win and not become addicted. They just walk away, taking their winnings with them, but a gambling addict cannot do this.

 HYPNOQUIT tips

Remove the temptation

These tips may seem pretty obvious, but it's amazing that when you are in the grip of an addiction you don't always think clearly and see the obvious.

- **Keep a journal** (see page 222): write down when the urge to gamble occurs and how you feel about the urge, at that time. Understand your triggers.
- **Cancel any subscriptions** you may have to gambling sites. Take your name off their lists.
- **Change your route home** if it normally takes you past the betting shop or casino, or a slot-machine arcade.
- **Keep busy**, distract your mind: get regular exercise, spend time with your family, take up a new hobby, visit relatives.
- **Promise yourself** to use the computer for work projects only (while *at work*) and never at home until you feel safe to do so.

HOW CAN HYPNOQUIT HELP YOU?

No matter how severe your gambling habit is, you can free yourself from this stressful and ruinous addiction. I know, because I've helped countless people do this.

Once you begin to do your daily meditations, listening to the CD and visualising yourself free from this addiction, you will quickly identify and break the subconscious connections that made you place those bets.

With Hypnoquit you will simply lose the urge to gamble – for ever. Your finances, relationships and quality of life will all start to improve dramatically.

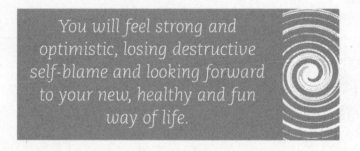

You will feel strong and optimistic, losing destructive self-blame and looking forward to your new, healthy and fun way of life.

Countless others have quitted their gambling addiction with my method. You can too!

Read Part 3, then use the action plan in Chapter 16 to get started.

PART 3

PREPARING FOR YOUR NEW LIFE

13

HOW LOVED ONES CAN HELP YOU

You have read this book accepting that you are dependent on something or controlled by a behaviour that you want to quit. It always helps to have the support of someone who loves and cares about you. This chapter is for them. To help you with your Hypnoquit programme I suggest you ask them to read this.

THE ADDICT'S PAIN

'Love the addict, hate the addiction.' This phrase is often used to help the loved ones of addicts, and it can be a useful way to look at the whole picture. Your loved one is in pain, but their behaviour ensures that you are in pain too. They may seem like a stranger at times. You may feel that you dislike them – that you don't even recognise them any more.

Addictions are incredibly complex and your role is complex too. In this chapter I am going to unravel the complexities to help you avoid taking on the negativity or guilt that your loved one feels, because you may be thinking, *Did I do something wrong to cause this addiction?*

HOW TO RECOGNISE AN ADDICT

An addict feels that they need their 'hit' just to survive. If they are forced to choose between a loved one and the addiction, they are compelled to choose the addiction, even though their heart may be telling them differently. An addict's judgement is impaired and they think they are being clever in hiding it; however, loved ones recognise how they've changed, because they adopt a defined pattern of behaviour as the addiction assumes greater importance in their daily life. Importantly, they haven't stopped loving those close to them, but this powerful addiction has taken hold of them.

Secrecy and lies

Many addicts will lie, deceive and manipulate those they love in order to continue with and fund their addictive behaviour. Giving up the addiction is terrifying for them, because in doing so they may have to face pain or insecurity, or other emotional issues that caused the addiction in the first place.

I always advise the loved ones of addicts to be supportive and not judgemental. I fully understand that you may be disappointed or angry, but anger and disapproval will not help either of you. Yes, secrecy and lies are part of the territory, but an addicted person is not enjoying him or herself. They probably did at the outset, but when they get to the stage of asking for help, the pain and anguish has invariably taken a front seat. It is undoubtedly foremost in their minds.

If you have read any of the other chapters in this book you

will see that there are many reasons why your loved one became addicted. An important factor is that sometimes an addict is in this situation because of the disappointment, disapproval or disinterest by mentors in their lives during childhood. This could come from parents, teachers, contemporaries or friends. As someone who cares, you don't want to mirror that behaviour, so it's wise to be prepared about how your own feelings might manifest themselves.

You probably feel pretty miffed to have to pick up the pieces; possibly you have done this before and you feel let down, yet again. But addiction is a condition just like any other, and it needs support.

> *Continue to love and support the person who is dear to you and needs to quit addiction, and you will be rewarded by helping them to achieve the best possible outcome for all concerned.*

WHAT YOU CAN DO

You no doubt agonise over what you should or shouldn't be doing and you may feel lost, inadequate and think it should be left to the professionals to sort out. To an extent this is absolutely correct; however, you can help too, and it will make your loved one's recovery easier for you as well. You will feel less excluded in the recovery and will begin to understand more about the addiction.

Here are some pointers to help you. Many people may

already be familiar with the following advice and decide to read this chapter as a refresher. Others, however, will be completely new to this game and may feel helpless. I hope you will find the following useful.

ACCEPT YOUR LIMITATIONS

You can't force an addict to get help. Essentially, the addict has to first recognise that they have a problem, secondly to admit it and finally to want help. You can support them and be there for them when they decide to quit, but you can't force them.

ARE YOU AN ENABLER?

Sometimes loved ones inadvertently become enablers – covering up for their addict, filling in the gaps, providing funds, making excuses for them and picking up the pieces. If this is you, I understand why you would do this: you love them and you want to protect them. It is probably the first time in your life that you have come across addictions, and you may assume your loved one must be weak or bad, or influenced by unsavoury friends.

You will be helping your loved one if you don't enable them anymore. If you stop throwing that lifeline out to them, they are more likely to realise that they need to quit far sooner than if you enable them to continue – to survive – while feeding their addiction.

In certain addictions this may involve watching your loved one hit rock bottom. This is horrendously painful for everyone concerned, but in the long term you will realise that you are actually doing them a huge favour. It won't seem that way at the time, that's for sure, and you may be in pain watching them. You may feel that you have to give in, but that would not help. If they have got this far, they can carry on to the final hurdle, and each day will get easier. Otherwise, if you do 'help' by giving in, he or she will have to go through all this pain again one day in order to quit.

With Hypnoquit the recovery is far less painful and sometimes there is no pain at all. This, of course, will depend on many factors including the particular addiction.

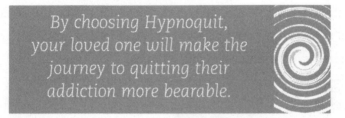

By choosing Hypnoquit, your loved one will make the journey to quitting their addiction more bearable.

KNOW YOUR BOUNDARIES, AND SET YOUR BOUNDARIES

You may begin to feel exploited and manipulated, and you will almost certainly feel anxious, angry, hurt and despairing at times. The best approach is to establish for yourself exactly what you will, and will not, accept. Set your boundaries. Let your loved one know what your boundaries are, very clearly in a loving way. But, above all, stick to them – always be consistent. They need consistency as much as you do and they need your continued love and support.

★ **Case Study:** Helen, 23, was using a mixture of drugs.
   Before treatment:
   Helen had been using a mixture of drugs since the age of 17. She said her parents' divorce was the catalyst, and she remembered as a child sitting on the top of the stairs most nights listening to them fight.

Helen's mum was self-employed in a cash business, and there was always cash around the house, so Helen began to steal it to fund her addiction. Her mum assumed it was Helen's less-than-desirable friends. She was aware that Helen was troubled and had become increasingly arrogant and stroppy, and difficult to live with. She also suspected her daughter was using drugs, but had no proof and was shocked when she discovered the extent of the problem. It certainly never occurred to her that it might be her own daughter stealing from her.

Eventually, valuables – jewellery, a laptop and ornaments – were going missing at an alarming rate and this was the final straw, so Helen's mum reluctantly set a trap and, to her horror, confirmed it was Helen after all. Although it was painful, her mum asked Helen to leave.

Helen moved in with her boyfriend and the same pattern continued. He was less tolerant and soon sent her packing, back to mum.

Helen had hit rock bottom and her mum was in despair to see her beautiful daughter, only 22, a college dropout, with nowhere to live, no job, and an addiction, so she had little choice but to take Helen back. But she did so with strict conditions for living at home: no stealing, no drugs and Helen had to get help. If Helen broke these rules, she was out. Helen was resentful of the rules but gradually began to understand and realise the pain she'd caused her mum and was ready to quit. She wanted to be clean more than anything.

After treatment:

Helen threw herself into Hypnoquit and turned her life around, putting her addiction behind her. She is now 23, is going back into education and has a new boyfriend. Her relationship with her mum has never been better.

HYPNOQUIT tips

'How can I help?'

- **Recognise that you can't 'cure' an addict.** Nothing you can say or do will stop your loved one from their addiction until they are ready to quit and seek help. It has to come from them.
- **Don't give up hope.** It's difficult, but your positive attitude can make a difference to how you both deal with their recovery.
- **Become informed.** The Internet, books and support groups can give you a lot of information that will help you to understand the nature of your loved one's addiction, and also your own situation and needs.
- **Don't enable.** Don't give them money or cover up for them.
- **Try not to judge.** This may be easier said than done, but if you can accept that your loved one is in pain and desperately needs your love and support, you will save yourself a lot of anguish.
- **Don't make them feel like a criminal.** They have a condition that needs help, and your love and support is equally important as the treatment itself.

'How can I protect myself?'

- **Set boundaries.** Work out what *you* will and won't accept from your loved one. Stick to the boundaries you have set; they are your survival bible.

> • **Get support.** You need support as much as the addict.
> Organisations for loved ones provide vital networks and support
> groups. These can seem like a lifeline for you at times. Or talk to
> a trusted non-critical friend or family member, if you prefer.

★ **Case Study:** Jenny is the mother of Dan, 22, who was a
cannabis addict.

Before treatment:

Jenny was desperate to get help for her son, to stop him
smoking cannabis, as he was becoming withdrawn,
paranoid and quick to fly into a temper. Her son was
changing from the gentle, happy, loving soul that she once
knew. Jenny's pain was raw and she was in turmoil. She
blamed herself for being so lenient when Dan was growing
up. Being a single mum, she felt the need to make up for his
absent father and would indulge him in every way possible.

I explored ways to help Jenny control her feelings and
anxieties. She had mixed emotions and felt that her son
was taking her for granted at times. She desperately
wanted to be loved by Dan. His father had rejected her, and
she didn't want her son to do the same. She felt that by
always giving in to his increasing demands, she would be
thought of as a perfect mother.

Day after day she returned home after a hard day's
work to be confronted with chaos and mess: a house full of
her son's friends, all smoking dope. Her son was oblivious
to her feelings and suffering. When she reached breaking
point and began yelling at him, he claimed she didn't
understand him.

Following the many arguments, Dan could dull his senses with cannabis but Jenny had nothing to relieve her pain. Family and friends urged tough love and to throw him out, but she could never contemplate that, whatever the circumstances. She stopped seeing them, as they might judge her precious Dan, and so she became more isolated herself – not because she wanted to, or because she had done anything to warrant this, but because of her son's addiction. Her inner strength and resolve enabled Jenny to stand by him and to cope with the situation, which seemed to be escalating out of control in Jenny's mind and she was becoming afraid for the future.

Dan overheard his mum sobbing one day and this was enough to make him realise how much he was hurting her – his mum, who had given her life to bring him up on her own – and Dan felt he had let her down badly. He saw a TV programme about someone in a similar situation to his own and, coupled with upsetting his mum, this was the catalyst he needed to seek help.

After treatment:
Hypnoquit delivered more than he could dream of. Dan quit his addiction very quickly. This was enough to make Jenny peaceful and happy again.

IT'S A HARD ROAD TO TRAVEL BUT WORTH IT

In short, loving and supporting an addict is never straightforward or easy. You may feel at times that you can't go on; you're in a corner, with nowhere to turn. You may also be feeling regrets, guilt or self-blame. But looking backwards is not helpful. Whatever has happened in the past, however much you feel you may – or, most likely, may not – have contributed to your loved one's addiction, you have to put that aside and move on.

Now is the time to do what you can, to support and help them. They may push you beyond all limits of tolerance and love while you do this, but set your boundaries, and stick with them.

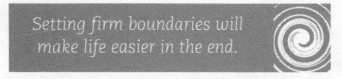

Setting firm boundaries will make life easier in the end.

Equally important, remember you are not alone, as there is always someone out there to help you and support you, but you have to ask, to make someone aware that you need help, love and comfort too.

There are countless people just like you. People who find themselves ripped apart by the addiction of a loved one. So, reach out, get support for yourself, and be determined. You can do this.

14

YOUR DELETE BUTTON

There was once a time in your life when you were not an addict. A time when there was no anxiety, guilt or stress surrounding the substance, and no behaviour to which you had become addicted. You were just yourself, free, possibly dipping into it now and again, but never hooked.

I'm going to help you to find the moment when all this changed for you. I am going to enable you to locate this moment, and then, quite literally, to delete it from your subconscious mind using the meditations on the CD.

By doing this, it's possible to erase any emotional complexities that caused you to turn to your addiction. You can then move forward into a new and straightforward way of life, one that will stay with you for ever.

I know this sounds unlikely, but it really does work. I've seen it happen in countless people whose addictions went back many years and their lives were painful and complicated, just like Oliver, overleaf.

★ **Case Study:** Oliver, 20, was addicted to alcohol and recreational drugs.

Before treatment:

'I was a very serious child and teenager and demanded a lot of attention. I was immature and needy, and my busy parents often screamed at me. I was always jealous of my two brothers, who my parents treated differently to me, more tolerantly, more loving. I had a few friends but no one really close, and deep down I was miserable. I lacked confidence and self-esteem and often my thoughts gave way to despair and feelings of anger, jealousy and depression. I masked all of this by playing the joker. I desperately needed to be accepted, to be liked and to feel normal and, importantly, to feel loved. At times my inadequacies and fears were so immense that I became almost suicidal. The resentment of an unhappy childhood welled up inside me, but above all there was fear – almost a fear of life.

'Then I got lucky and I discovered drink and drugs! I even found a new friend, Pete, and we became inseparable. Pete introduced me to a new way of life! This was the moment when everything changed for me: my first sip of booze, aged 15. Drink and drugs gave my life a whole new meaning. They changed the way I felt inside. When I felt unhappy, alcohol would fix it. When I felt inadequate, a joint or line of cocaine would calm me down and boost my confidence.

'Of course it didn't last. All my despair, frustrations and fears came flooding back and intensified many times over. But now there were other feelings too: shame, paranoia, self-loathing, damaged pride and feelings of guilt. Dependency hadn't worked. It was a living hell.

'After five years of addiction I had reached the depths of

*despair, but this time fear actually saved me. It wasn't a fear
of my parents finding out or my brothers ridiculing me. It
was the fear of death, as Pete had died from a cocktail of
alcohol and drug overdose, and I was devastated to lose
him.'*

After treatment:

Oliver told me months later, 'My road to recovery all began
with Hypnoquit and our sessions together. You accepted me
for what I was and easily won my trust, helping me to be
aware of my feelings, and to accept and understand them.
You showed you cared. Overall, my recovery from addiction
was so much easier than I thought it would be.

'I began to understand that my childhood wasn't as
unhappy as it had become in my own mind. Of course, not
everything was a figment of my imagination, but most was
exaggerated. I realised my problems stemmed from jealousy
of my two brothers, who had come along when my father's
income had increased enormously, so they got more privileges
than I had when growing up. Also, my parents were focusing
on a new business venture when my brothers were young,
and so they were happier. We moved to a bigger house and
they were definitely more lenient with my brothers.

'So, while my parents seemed tough on me and soft on
my brothers, it wasn't their fault. More importantly, I realise
through hypnosis that it was a different set of circumstances
and not me that was unlovable.

'I do believe that I went down the road of destruction
with Pete to try to hurt my parents – and my brothers too, I
guess – to get some attention, to say "Hello, I am here too!"
Although I am very sad for Pete, we were very different

individuals and probably wouldn't have become close friends without the addictions.

'These days I feel happy and normal. I am no longer ruled by urges and cravings. I feel calm and healthy and much more aware of my emotions, much more "in the moment". I feel like the cause of my addiction has simply been found, and switched off.'

MORE THAN JUST A MOMENT

Of course, it's often not quite as simple as identifying an instant where everything changed for you – or to find a reason for your addiction. Indeed, it can sometimes feel that the 'moment' when your attitude changed is actually way more than a moment; it's an entire period of your life. With this programme you don't even need to be consciously aware of the moment when it all changed for you. This is because I work with your subconscious mind. I reprogram your thought processes, via your subconscious urges, so that you can put your addiction behind you – for good.

LOCATING THAT DELETE BUTTON

My approach is personal to you. While writing this book, I always proofread aloud to myself so that I can put myself into the reader's shoes and feel what you may be feeling. As I read through, I feel, once again, the emotions of the day I encountered Oliver, or the many people I see every day in my consulting rooms in London's Harley Street or elsewhere in the world.

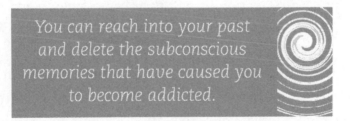

*You are my personal client,
and I want you to succeed.*

I am immensely passionate about my work and I want this passion to come through to you, so that you feel that I want to, and will, help you in the same passionate way that I have helped Oliver and all my other clients, whether you are in my consulting rooms or reading this book and then listening to the CD.

You *can* find the answer

Hypnoquit works with or without therapy, whether face-to-face or through reading my book and listening to the CD. It can help you to reach back to a time before these complexities began.

*You can reach into your past
and delete the subconscious
memories that have caused you
to become addicted.*

Of course, not everyone will be able to automatically pinpoint a moment when it all changed. You may think that your childhood is far too complicated to pick through. You may worry that your problems with addiction are so deep-seated that you'll never work out where it all started.

Equally, you may well think that your addiction is not complicated at all. You just love alcohol, or gambling, or food, or sex, or drugs, but to excess! People often say this to me, and I tell them that if they are consistently indulging, they cannot stop themselves and it interferes with their everyday life and relationships, as well as occupying too much thinking time, and they feel guilty, then there is a problem.

Note

If you enjoy alcohol, or gambling, or food, sex or drugs seemingly more than average – more than your friends or colleagues – but it doesn't control your life, then you simply have a good appetite for life's indulgences.

HOW DO YOU FIND YOUR DELETE BUTTON?

Using the meditations on the CD, you will be able to reach a state of deep relaxation. It will then be possible to access the moment when it all changed, before you became addicted. Don't worry, I will help you to find that moment. Even though you may not be able to put your finger on the cause in your normal waking consciousness, the delete button is there and can be found during your meditations. What's more, you will find it during your first meditation.

> *The good news: we all have a delete button. You have a time before you became addicted. Hypnoquit will help you to find this time and to press that button.*

Here's how to use your delete button:

1 **Relax and go back.** As you listen to the accompanying CD you will enter a relaxed hypnotic state. I will then guide you to a place where you were free before your addiction.

2 **Find your turning point.** When did that time change? I will look for a transitional period in your life: when you started to become compelled to indulge more and more; when you started to lose the pleasure, and feel more and more compulsion. I will help you to find that point through hypnosis on the CD, and then I will delete it.

3 **Keep the feeling.** I will bring the feeling of this transitional period in your life to the moment when the addiction began, to the forefront of your mind.

4 **Press delete.** I will delete the emotional associations and complexities. As I've mentioned before, this is just like deleting files from a computer. These are defective files; you don't need them any more. I will help you to remove all the emotional associations that trigger your addiction, whether they are for comfort, or because of boredom, stress or tiredness.

◎ HYPNOQUIT tip
Let me make it easy for you

Don't worry! I will guide you and we will work together. The beauty of Hypnoquit is that I will guide you through your past, and you will not find it anxiety provoking.

LET YOUR SUBCONSCIOUS WORK

The beauty of hypnosis is that you don't need to know, consciously, when your addiction began. The subconscious mind knows everything about you. It is where you store all your experiences and past emotions. When you are in the state of deep relaxation – hypnosis – I am speaking directly to your subconscious mind. It knows exactly where that button is and will delete it as directed by me. It really is as simple as that.

Of course, I'm not saying that the emotions just vanish into thin air. They are still in your subconscious somewhere. So you will still be able to recall your period of addiction but will not have the same attachment to it, as the addiction will have gone. But the point is that once the connection is deleted, these emotions will no longer influence your habits. This is what I mean by pressing your delete button.

Hypnosis can change your mind

Although hypnosis is surrounded in mystery, it should not be. It is simply the power of the mind: I change your negative thoughts into positive ones. You may think you cannot achieve a task, such as giving up smoking, or cutting out alcohol, because you have been indoctrinated and weaned on that fact for years. Hypnosis enables those changes to happen.

Often my clients say to me, 'I don't know what you have done or how you do it, but it's as though you have somehow short-circuited my brain and reprogrammed me to do the things I want to do and have been unable to do. Yet I now do them without even trying.' That is how you will be too.

You don't have to relive the agony

I don't want you to relive your past experiences, as they may be painful, although not necessarily so.

It's all learned behaviour

When a child is continually told that they are clumsy, sure enough, that child will grow into adulthood not so gracefully: stepping on people's toes, dropping things and bumping into people and objects – that is, until they are reprogrammed to believe that they are not clumsy at all. After all, they were not born clumsy, they have just learned to be, because they have been told continually that is what they are.

Any learned behaviour – such as eating disorders, sexual behaviour, gambling, drug taking, drinking or smoking – works this way too. **A person is not born an addict; they learn to be one.**

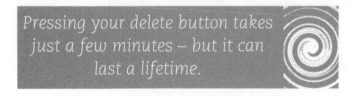

Pressing your delete button takes just a few minutes – but it can last a lifetime.

KEEPING THE MESSAGE STRONG

Hypnosis is always effective, and practising your daily meditations with the CD will reinforce the message. This needs to be just 'topped up' once or twice each week after you are confident your addiction is behind you, to keep the message in the forefront of your mind. For some addictions, such as smoking, you may only need to listen to the CD once. Once you feel comfortable that your addiction is over, you will no longer need to listen to the CD, but it is always there if you feel tempted.

WHAT HAPPENS NOW?

From now on, you will be free from your addiction. You will not turn to it when you need comfort or love, or because you feel anxious or stressed, you will find comfort and love in other more fulfilling and constructive ways. Your positive mental attitude will enable you to find ways to deal with anxious or stressed moments. The delete button is a powerful tool. It's time to find yours and press it!

15

REPROGRAM YOUR MIND

Your self-hypnosis meditations are immensely powerful. They will not only help you to kick your addiction but they'll also help you to live a longer, healthier life and to develop a positive, focused and happy outlook.

I am often asked how to get the most from the daily meditation time. It is certainly possible to maximise the impact of your reprogramming meditations. So, this is how you do it:

PREPARE FOR YOUR MEDITATION

1 **Set aside about 20 minutes each day** until you are no longer addicted. You may feel a need, or simply want, to listen to the CD just once or twice a week to maintain freedom from addiction. Find a regular time that suits you, and make your meditation a part of your life.
2 **Find a quiet spot** away from distractions. Don't be over-concerned about background noise though, you don't need absolute silence.
3 **Have your Visualisation Tool** handy (see page 214).
4 **Have your CD ready** to start playing, or you may have downloaded it onto your iPod.

5 **Focus on your Visualisation Tool** before closing your eyes.

6 **Now begin the meditation,** following my instructions.

USE YOUR VISUALISATIONS

You want to be free from addiction. But what does this actually mean? It is vital to have a clear goal from the outset. It's actually no good just saying, 'I want to be a non-smoker.' Or 'I want to stop craving alcohol/food/gambling/sex/drugs.' I want you to be far more specific than that. Being specific involves visualising your new self in detail: building a three-dimensional, vivid picture of yourself when you have kicked your addiction.

What does it feel like to be the new you?

To create an effective change, you first have to work out exactly what being free from addiction means – to you. It's important to produce a clear picture of your future self: how does this new you look, feel, and behave? To do this properly, you need to develop a skill called 'visualisation'. Visualisation will become an important part of your daily meditations. To help your visualisations you will need to make a Visualisation Tool, which is simply a picture of yourself free from addictions. It will also contain positive affirmations to help reinforce the encouraging words that you will hear from me during the meditations.

EXERCISE: create a Visualisation Tool

1 Find a photograph of yourself before you became addicted, when you were happy and healthy. People often find it helpful to make a collage with their photograph in

the centre. Write affirmations – positive and meaningful statements – about what you will achieve in your addiction-free future around the photo. Keep the collage small and compact, so that you can keep it with you.

2   Your Visualisation Tool will give you a far more vivid goal. It will put the image of the new you into your subconscious, so that you genuinely believe that it's possible for you to become that person, to become addiction-free.

3   Visualisations are a key reminder, throughout the day, of your goal. You can look at your Visualisation Tool at any time to help you continue on your path to recovery.

Here are some examples of affirmations that you might find helpful:

'I close my eyes and think positive and loving thoughts.'
'Today I am taking control of my life.'
'I am in control of my own thoughts and I am confident to be addiction-free.'
'I love myself completely, so I know I can give love to others.'
'I deserve to live an addiction-free life.'
'I will let go of my fears as I enter happily into an addiction-free life.'

You will find more affirmations in Chapter 16.

HYPNOQUIT tip

Build a mental picture

If you can't find a photo, cast your mind back to a time when you felt happy, positive and addiction-free. Picture your future self this way: addiction-free, happy and enjoying life again.

This process and your Visualisation Tool will be a vital part of your recovery.

How to use your Visualisation Tool

Use your Visualisation Tool as part of your daily meditations while listening to the CD. Here's how:

1 Each time you listen to the CD, take a moment to look at and study your Visualisation Tool, your collage. Really focus on it for a few moments, before closing your eyes. When you get to the section in the CD where I ask you to imagine yourself, as you want to be, you will have that image clearly in your mind. You'll see how easy this is.

2 Listen to the CD every day and see this as part of your daily routine. You'll be amazed at how quickly and easily you reach this dream state. The fact is, it's not a dream, it's a reality – *your* reality.

How to build on your visualisations

1 **Deepen your visualisation.** Think about how you'll feel when you are no longer addicted. You want to be 'clean' or 'free' or 'normal', but what does this actually mean to you? Take your time to think, and be specific with yourself about how you will feel to be free from your addiction.

- How much better do you want to feel?
- How will your friends and family see you?
- How will you see yourself?
- What physical changes will you notice – your skin, hair, teeth?

- What emotional changes will there be?
- How will you feel inside?

2 **Use mini-visualisations** (see below). You can use this skill whenever you find yourself sitting or standing around waiting. It will help to reinforce your meditations.

HYPNOQUIT tip

Keep remembering

Make your Visualisation Tool relatively small. Keep it handy – somewhere you can access it regularly: your handbag or wallet, or slotted inside your daily diary. You'll then be reminded visually of your goal, throughout the day and in any moments of weakness in the early days of becoming addiction-free.

Mini-visualisations

You can use your visualisation skills any time in addition to your daily meditations – while waiting for a bus, in the GP surgery, or simply when you're feeling bored. Mini-visualisations are a good way to constantly remind yourself where you are heading, to your addiction-free future, and what it means to you and why. This only takes a moment:

1 Take a look at your Visualisation Tool if you have it with you, or picture it in your mind.

2 Slow your breathing. Close your eyes, take a deep breath in through your nose and deep into your lungs. Fill your lungs with oxygen. Hold for a moment, and then slowly release the breath through your mouth. Repeat this deep breathing in and out about ten times. Each time you

breathe in, fill your lungs with more oxygen. Regular breathing exercises help you to breathe correctly, so this is a good skill to have anyway.

3   Take a moment to visualise your addiction-free self. Think of all the benefits this will bring. Picture your Visualisation Tool. This will help to reinforce the work you are doing to help you quit your addiction. Your instant reaction may be: 'That's impossible!' But I can assure you it isn't. I have helped thousands of people just like you to realise that 'impossibility' and I am going to help you, too.

4   Enter, mindfully, into your new identity: what do I see when I look in the mirror? How does it feel to live in this new, healthy body? You are not afraid to let go of your addiction. You embrace it.

5   Enjoy the new you!

THE NEW YOU

This might all sound ridiculous, but most people have very visual brains. It is enormously powerful to be able to 'see' your recovered self, to genuinely believe that it is possible for you to become that person, to become addiction-free.

Many people initially find this part of the programme difficult to get their heads around. They think, *This won't work for me* or *I'll never be that way*. You will! Don't give up. Your daily meditation and visualisations both take practice, but they will become a vital part of your recovery. You will very quickly realise that Hypnoquit is here to change your life, to spin you around, turn you upside down – if you like – and back on your feet again.

Think about all the extra time that you will have for your

family, friends and hobbies when you are back in the real world again. You will be able to feel life, to feel love. Addictions can take this away from you when you are in the addiction zone.

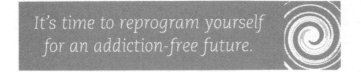

It's time to reprogram yourself for an addiction-free future.

I've worked with many people who have overcome their doubts, and made the meditations and visualisations really work for them. These people have turned their lives around and have lost their addiction for ever. Think of all the time and mental energy you currently waste thinking about and being involved in your addiction. From now on all that energy can be used for other, far more important, things. For yourself for starters.

Clients of mine have changed careers, taken up activities they'd always wanted to try, ended or begun relationships or thrown themselves into new projects – all kick-started by Hypnoquit.

Your meditations and visualisations are just the start. It's time to reprogram yourself for a new you and a new future. Make them work for you!

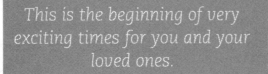

This is the beginning of very exciting times for you and your loved ones.

Chapter 16 contains your action plan for quitting addiction. Read through that to familiarise yourself with what you need to prepare in advance and how the programme works in practice. Afterwards, read Chapter 17 while you focus your mind on this new exciting step towards your life without addiction.

16

YOUR HYPNOQUIT ACTION PLAN

'Ve explained how addictions take hold and you should now have a better understanding of what your addictions are and how they are affecting your life. I have also explained earlier in this Part 3 how loved ones can help you, and I have described the role of visualisations and how, through the Hypnoquit meditations, I will press your delete button to reprogram your mind. Are you now ready to start using Hypnoquit to free yourself of your addiction's control? If you are ready, and you're certain that you are doing this for you alone, this chapter will guide you through. If you don't feel quite ready, revisit my suggestion of completing an addiction diary on page 18.

GET SUPPORT

Don't forget that support from your loved one will help you to reach your goal. Ask them to read Chapter 13.

GET READY

There are just a few things you need to prepare in advance, then you're ready to go. It's especially important to take the time to create your Visualisation Tool so that it's just the way you want it to be, as it will give you the inspiration for continuing success.

1 **Make your Visualisation Tool.** See Chapter 15 for how to do this. If you are a food addict, there is specific advice for you on page 84.
2 **Record the meditation CD** onto your iPod or MP3 player, if you like, so that you can continue to meditate each day, even if you are away from home.
3 **Have an exercise book or journal** ready as explained overleaf (also see page 81 for the food diary or page 159 for the alcohol diary).

PRACTISING MINDFULNESS

For those of you who are new to mindfulness, by living in a mindful way you give your full attention to the present moment rather than focusing on the past or the future. Through mindfulness, you will undoubtedly enjoy life far more and will learn to live more calmly. You will learn to live in the 'now' and this will help you to easily distance yourself from the cravings and triggers which caused your addiction. Keeping your daily journal will make you more mindful of everything you are doing and will enable you to keep your focus on the present and monitor how well you are progressing in taking control of your life.

KEEPING YOUR JOURNAL

Use a small notebook for your journal and one that is small enough to pop into your bag or your pocket so that it's always with you. Use two pages for each day and record your daily activities on one page and your emotions and behaviour on the other. Each day, after you have listened to your CD, write 'CD' in the top right-hand corner of that day's page.

As you complete each day's entries, you will begin to see a pattern emerging: you will start to see a correlation between the two entries: your feelings and your actions. You will also see, and be able to chart, your progress in quitting your addiction. See pages 46–8 for an example of a completed journal.

If you are a food addict, remember to fill in your food diary as described on page 81. This is an essential part of the programme and you will gain great benefits from completing it. Remember also to eat mindfully as described on pages 73–4, so that you really enjoy and appreciate every mouthful.

If you are drinking too much alcohol, remember to fill in your alcohol diary as described on page 159. This will help you to see at a glance how much you are drinking and it will help to spur you on to making changes.

With all addictions, your daily journal will help you to see how often you indulge in your particular addiction and how your emotions have an effect. You can then use this information to tackle your addiction.

Affirmations

One of the cornerstones of my daily meditation CD is making affirmations. This means repeating a simple sentence that will reinforce a positive mindset. Rest assured that the long-term effects of addiction can be overcome. Addiction exists in the mind, even when there is a physical component. So, you must change the way you think: re-educate your thought processes. The fastest way to do this is with hypnosis and using affirmations such as, 'I am freeing myself from guilt and shame' and 'I love myself'. Having such an affirmation to repeat to yourself frequently helps the recovery process enormously.

I'm going to ask you to build affirmations into your meditations and to use them in quiet – or stressful – moments to reinforce the new you. Here are some affirmations I often suggest to clients but, by all means, develop your own simple, easy-to-remember, meaningful ones:

- I am loveable.
- I am decisive and self-assured, and confident that I will succeed.
- I love and accept every part of myself.
- I am worthy of love and respect.
- My life has real meaning and purpose.
- I accept full responsibility for my recovery.
- Every day I am getting better and better, stronger and stronger.
- I feel whole as a person, and I love myself.
- I will succeed and remain successful.
- My approach is positive, and I will remain positive.

- My [eating/shopping/drinking etc.] does not define me or make me happier, I am me and proud of myself.

You will hear some affirmations when you listen to the CD and you can see a list of a few more in Chapter 15.

Build some affirmations into your daily CD meditations, and you will find your past addicted self just melting away and a strong, focused new you will emerge from within.

You can overcome whatever caused your addiction; you can take back control and move on with your life. You can become healthy and positive, leaving that addiction far behind you as a distant memory.

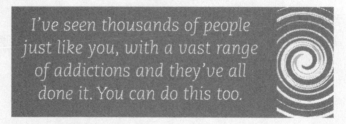

I've seen thousands of people just like you, with a vast range of addictions and they've all done it. You can do this too.

PREPARE FOR THE MEDITATION

Here is a reminder to get you started on the meditations – the essential part of the Hypnoquit programme:

1 **Set aside about 20 minutes each day** to listen to your CD until you are no longer addicted. You may feel a need, or simply want, to listen to the CD just once or twice a week to maintain freedom from addiction. Find a regular time that suits you, and make your meditation a part of your life.

2 **Find a quiet spot** away from distractions. Don't be over-concerned about background noise though, you don't need absolute silence.
3 **Have your Visualisation Tool** handy.
4 **Have your CD ready** to start playing, or you may have downloaded it onto your iPod.
5 **Focus on your Visualisation Tool** before closing your eyes.
6 **Now begin the meditation**, following my instructions.

Your visualisations picture your goal

Remember that your visualisations will give you a clear picture of yourself addiction-free. That is the person you will very soon become: clear from addiction, happy and free from the worries, cost and ill health that has been your past.

USING YOUR CD

Listen to your CD every day. (It's OK to miss out the occasional day.) When you are free of your addiction, play the CD just twice a week to maintain your resolve. Listening to the CD is pleasantly relaxing and empties your mind of all the day's irrelevancies, and it calms and centres you and stills the mind. This is the core of Hypnoquit.

Feel the benefit from the very first meditation.

Some people find that listening to the CD once only is enough to conquer a particular addiction, such as smoking. For others, it will require listening to the CD repeatedly to get the same effect. This depends on two major factors. Firstly, your particular addiction, as some addictions do require more re-inforcement. Secondly, your strong desire to quit your habit rather than just thinking that it would be a good idea. But do remember that as long as you want to quit for you alone, then you will be able to do so.

Your daily planner

- Add to your journal throughout the day. It helps you to practise mindfulness.
- Decide on a regular time to listen to the CD – it could be in the morning before you go to work, or during the evening, or just before you go to bed. Make this the same time every day if possible and at a time when you will not fall asleep while listening to the CD. It is important to be aware, pleasantly relaxed, but aware.
- Think about the affirmations that appeal to you.
- Say your affirmations quietly to yourself (and at any time throughout the day).
- Enjoy the new-found confidence you have gained through freeing yourself of your addiction.

BUILD ON YOUR MEDITATIONS

Now you're getting into the swing of the meditations, think about how you can get more out of them.

1 After you have used the CD a few times, deepen your visualisation, if you like, by following my tip on page 216.

2 Use my mini-visualisation on page 217 whenever you are just sitting or standing around waiting to remind yourself of your happier life without addiction.

> *As the days go by, you'll be feeling a great sense of achievement.*

Exercise will help you

Try to factor in some exercise each day. Just a 20-minute walk can revitalise you and make you feel more relaxed. Exercise is something that you may have forgotten about while you focused on your addiction – make it a part of your life today.

Now, read my final chapter before you begin the Hypnoquit programme.

17

LIFE STARTS HERE

You should now have a clear idea of how hypnosis works on your mind and what Hypnoquit can do for you. Hypnoquit can bring dramatic changes to your life, benefiting the way you look after yourself, and its principles can become a natural part of your everyday life.

Hypnoquit is a mind-changing revolution: a simple self-hypnosis technique that will free you from your addictive behaviour, for ever. It works because it removes the guilt, anxiety and stress associated with addictions. It is a simple yet radical way to gain control of your life without therapy or soul-searching.

Most addicts feel despair, while their self-esteem and self-worth plummets. They feel they will never get control. Hypnoquit offers a way out that is simple and effective. It has helped thousands of addicts, just like you, to quit this destructive behaviour for good.

Addiction can take many forms, and it can be incredibly obvious – or incredibly well hidden. It is hugely destructive, affecting not just your life but also the lives of those around you.

Most people with addictions already know what they have to do in order to quit, but it all seems too difficult.

> *Hypnoquit can liberate anyone from addictions. It is a way to gain control of your life, to recapture your self-confidence and to rebuild healthy and normal relationships with those close to you.*

As you will remember from Chapter 3, I explained that the concept of mindfulness is central to Hypnoquit. Mindfulness is gathering force as a highly effective psychological tool, both in popular culture and mainstream psychology. It shows you how to mindfully conquer your addictive behaviour, making life-enhancing choices. In short, Hypnoquit helps you to kick the habit, from the inside out – from the mind itself.

> *You will quickly start to enjoy life again, make long-lasting and life-enhancing decisions to change your relationship with your addiction, change your behaviour, and stay there for life.*

Once you have started Hypnoquit and enjoyed all the freedom it brings, you will find that it's easy to live addiction-free, because that is what you will want to do. It won't be a hassle, and you won't feel guilt any more or be depressed. You will thrive on the success you are achieving day by day. It will be a part of your life. Simply by making your meditations a regular habit and following my basic recommendations, addictions will be a thing of the past. Healthy addiction-free living will be your present and your future.

Now, I hope, you know what you are aiming for when it comes to planning an addiction-free life ahead. Beginning a healthy lifestyle is straightforward and inspiring when you use the guidance of the meditations on the CD.

FIND CONFIDENCE NOW IN YOUR ADDICTION-FREE FUTURE

You will start to feel the changes in your behaviour and attitude as soon as you have had your first Hypnoquit meditation. Hypnoquit promotes a mindful awareness to change your attitude towards addictions – *and it works instantly*. As you continue with the programme you will see many more changes over the coming days and weeks.

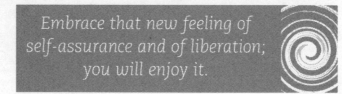

Embrace that new feeling of self-assurance and of liberation; you will enjoy it.

In short, you will feel empowered by your new addiction-free self and your new-found confidence.

SUCCESS IS JUST AROUND THE CORNER

You no longer need to feel trapped in an addiction, which has taken you out of the realms of society at times, and which made you feel so unhappy, and even angry. Now you can join the many people who have turned their lives around as they lose their preoccupation with their addiction.

You will be one of the many Hypnoquit success stories

Remember the words of past addicts you have discovered in this book, who have found a new life with Hypnoquit:

Colin: 'This has been so easy and I feel clean and healthy.'

Jennifer: 'I am surprised how this method has changed my whole concept of food and addictions and has given me more time to enjoy other things in my life, like family, friends and sport.'

Rachel: 'Hypnoquit helped me to turn my life around.'

Cassie: '[Hypnoquit] has also saved my marriage, but more importantly this method has saved, and probably salvaged, my children's lives.'

Andrea: 'I feel like a new person.'

Nancy: 'This programme not only helped me to come off the drugs but also to rediscover my inner strengths of self-confidence, self-esteem, self-worth and self-belief, and for that I am more than eternally grateful.'

Jim: 'I have my life back.'

Lisa: 'Hypnoquit isn't about looking back, or regrets, and I'm grateful for that – I'm happy and looking forward to the rest of my life.'

Oliver: 'I feel calm and healthy and much more aware of my emotions, much more "in the moment". I feel like the cause of my addiction has simply been found, and switched off.'

TIME TO MAKE IT HAPPEN

So, now it's over to you. Use my CD for your daily meditations and start writing in your daily journal. Re-read this book or selected chapters, whenever you want inspiration, ideas or clarification. You are now one of thousands of people who have turned their lives around with Hypnoquit.

It starts right here, right now. Enjoy it!

Index